POP

WHEN SPORT BRINGS US TO OUR KNEES

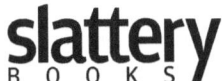

**Australian athletes share their
ACL injury journeys**

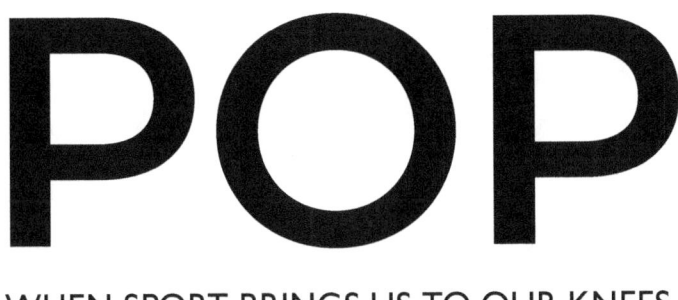

WHEN SPORT BRINGS US TO OUR KNEES

JESS CUNNINGHAM

Produced by the Slattery Media Group Pty Ltd for Jess Cunningham

JESS CUNNINGHAM
www.jesscunningham.com.au

Slattery Media Group Pty Ltd
902/31 Spring Street, Melbourne, 3000
slatterymedia.com

Text © Jess Cunningham 2022

First published by Jess Cunningham 2022

All rights reserved. No part of this publication may be reproduced, stored in a retrieval system or transmitted in any form or by any means without the prior written permission of the copyright owner. Inquiries should be made to the publisher.

 A catalogue record for this book is available from the National Library of Australia

ISBN: 978-0-6454913-0-2

Group Publisher: Geoff Slattery
Cover design: Alice Beattie
Typeset: Kate Slattery

Printed and bound in Australia by Ingram Spark Publishers

Written on Dharawal Country with acknowledgement and respect to the traditional owners of the lands and waterways upon which Australian sport is played

DEDICATION

To my clients and their knees

POP /pop/

Noun/verb - the sound or sensation often felt in the knee when an ACL injury occurs

Abbreviation of popularise – to make a scientific or academic subject accessible to the general public by presenting it in an understandable or relatable form

CONTENTS

PART 1
ABOUT THIS BOOK

We have an ACL problem xi
    What is the ACL? xiv
    The knee xiv
    ACL injury xv
    Diagnosis of an ACL injury xv
    What is an ACL reconstruction? xv
How to use this book xvi
A note from the author xviii

PART 2
ATHLETES' STORIES

Aerial skiing	Lydia Lassila	3
American football	Adam Gotsis	21
Football (soccer)	Lydia Williams	35
Netball	Kim Green	49
Rugby Union	Mitch Short	61
Freestyle skiing	Anna Segal	71
Australian Football	Daniel Menzel	85

CONTENTS

Snowboard cross	Belle Brockhoff	101
Rugby Union	Damien Fitzpatrick	115
Cricket	Callum Ferguson	131
Freestyle skiing	Russ Henshaw	143
Sailing	Eliza Solly	157
Ice Hockey	Nathan Walker	171

PART 3
AFTERWORD

Listen and learn 181
    ACL Cheat Sheet 182
Setting yourself up for success 184
Prevent, perform, recover, & reflect 184
    Sport specific programs for
        injury prevention 185
Learn, connect & share 187

Acknowledgements 188
Glossary 191
Endnotes 200

PART 1

ABOUT THIS BOOK

INTRODUCTION

WE HAVE AN ACL PROBLEM

There's no denying that Australia is a sports-loving nation. We punch well above our weight on the international stage and have a rich sporting culture. Whether playing, watching, or talking about sport, we really can't seem to get enough.

But our love of sport also seems to be bringing us to our knees.

Research has shown that in Australia we have the highest rate of anterior cruciate ligament reconstruction (ACLR) in the world.[1] Between 2000-2015, a total of 197,557 primary ACLRs were performed in Australia. During this time, the average incidence of ACLR increased by 43 per cent, and more alarmingly by 75 per cent in those under 25 years of age. Revision surgery also increased by 5.6 per cent per year. Direct hospital costs of ACLR surgery in 2014-2015 were estimated to be $142 million. We also know that females are up to six times more likely to injure their anterior cruciate ligament (ACL) compared to males due to differences in hormones, biomechanics, neuromuscular control,[2] and gendered social and cultural factors such as training access and training age. With stats like these, it is clear we need to look closely at how we approach the way we are managing and working to prevent ACL injuries.

Of course, prevention is always better than a cure. The first step in reducing our alarmingly high rates of ACLR surgery is to simply stop the injury from occurring in the first place. There are many evidence-based sports-specific ACL injury prevention programs that have been shown to reduce the likelihood of ACL and lower limb injury by around half in all athletes, and up to two-thirds in females[3,4,5] (see Part 3 for a full list of sport specific programs). As well as reducing injuries, these programs have the added benefit of improving performance and require only 10-15 minutes to complete—either before or after training and games, or at home.[6] For the programs to be effective they need to be completed routinely, and in an ideal world at all levels of sport. Yet a huge gap continues to exist between this knowledge and it's implementation. Increased public awareness as to the existence of these programs is required.

For those who suffer an ACL rupture, the automatic assumption and narrative surrounding the injury has historically been that surgery is required (it was thought that the torn ACL could not heal) and that the athlete's sporting season is over. But emerging research suggests we may need to rethink this approach[7] with spontaneous ACL healing shown to occur[8,9,10] in nearly two-thirds of full ACL ruptures[11]. Good results have also been obtained from non-surgical management and thorough rehabilitation.[12]

The sports medicine world has long known it is possible to manage without an ACL, and those who cope with its absence are not limited to leading sedentary lives as was often traditionally thought. There are growing examples of athletes returning to pivoting and high impact sports without an intact ACL;[13,14,15,16,17] who are not just surviving but thriving in their sport, as well as maintaining good knee function into the future.[18,19,20]

Despite these research findings, it must be stressed that not everyone is a 'coper', and that for some, ACLR remains the best option. ACL injury management must always be considered on an individual basis, with patients made aware of the surgical and non-surgical treatment options available and their similar outcomes regarding the risk of future meniscal tears and osteoarthritis.[21,22,23]

Regardless of which management option is sought, there can be no denying that ACL injury is a significant interruption to anyone's physical life and requires an involved period of rehabilitation if optimal physical performance is to be achieved. Although the timeframe for returning to sport is anything but exact, realistic expectations and the achievement of functional strength and ability milestones throughout the rehabilitation process is vital. However, unfortunately for many this is not always the case. Research shows that returning to sport before nine months post-ACLR is associated with up to a seven-times increased risk of re-rupture,[24] and worryingly most adolescents expect to return in six months or less,[25] with fewer than 15 per cent passing their return-to-sport clearance testing criteria at eight to nine months after surgery.[26,27] Obviously it is important to increase awareness around setting realistic expectations for return-to-sport timeframes, and the successful completion of end-stage rehab cannot be overlooked if the increasing rate of re-ruptures is to be reduced.

No matter how telling these research findings are, the fact is that most of us don't respond well to such data. And so there will be no further discussion in this book about statistics and numerical research findings. Instead, the pages are filled with what we respond to best—stories and emotions, all told by successful athletes from their lived experiences with ACL injury and rehabilitation.

The purpose of this book is not to argue whether conservative or surgical management is the better option, but rather to provide a valuable resource offering inspiration and education around the rehabilitation journey ahead for those who have suffered an ACL injury.

The common phrase heard from all the athletes interviewed for this book was, "I wish something like that had existed when I was going through it all."

Now it does.

WHAT IS THE ACL?

The ACL is one of the four main ligaments (a strong band of fibrous connective tissue connecting bone to bone) that connects the thigh bone (femur) to the shin bone (tibia). It runs diagonally—deep within the knee joint connecting the back of the femur to the front of the tibia—and forms a cross with the posterior cruciate ligament (PCL) which runs in the opposite direction, hence its name (cruciate is from the Latin word for cross). The ACL and the PCL work together to stabilise the knee during impact and rotational forces. The two other main ligaments—the medial collateral ligament (MCL) and lateral collateral ligament (LCL) run vertically on either side of the knee to support side to side movements.

THE KNEE

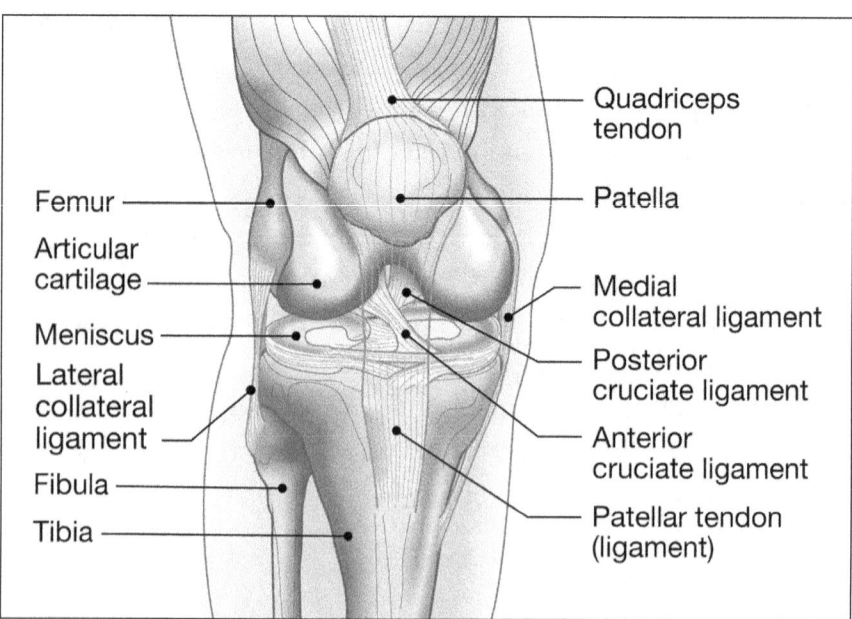

ACL INJURY

Rupturing the ACL is one of the most common knee sporting injuries and can occur from direct trauma (contact to the outside of the knee in a tackle), as a result of twisting force through the knee (cutting or pivoting movements to avoid an opponent), or from awkward landings (landing off-balance with more weight on one leg). Other structures such as the medial and lateral meniscus (shock absorbing crescents of cartilage between the tibia and femur) may or may not also be injured in the same movement.

DIAGNOSIS OF AN ACL INJURY

A tell-tale 'pop' is often felt or heard as the ligament fails. Swelling is usually immediate and significant. The integrity of the ACL is assessed most commonly using two main tests performed by clinicians—the Lachman's test and pivot shift test. Magnetic Resonance Imaging (MRI) is usually utilised to confirm the diagnosis.

WHAT IS AN ACL RECONSTRUCTION (ACLR)?

Management of an ACL rupture can either be surgical or conservative. When surgery is performed it aims to reconstruct the damaged ligament using a graft to restore the internal stability of the knee. The surgery is performed using a minimally invasive arthroscopic approach where surgical tools and a small camera are inserted into small incisions on either side of the knee.

The graft can be:

- an autograft (tissue from the person's own body—using the hamstring, patella tendon, quadriceps tendon);
- an allograft (tissue from a donor—cadaver Achilles);
- synthetic (a Ligament Augmentation and Reconstruction System (LARS) graft—note these are no longer commonly used due to poor outcomes).

HOW TO USE THIS BOOK

The intended purpose of this book is to share the journeys of athletes (both with, and without their ACLs) who have successfully returned to sport after an ACL injury, and to inspire and motivate individuals who are currently in rehab. I hope it can be a helpful tool that therapists and surgeons—and friends and family—can offer to the injured, whether they be professional or aspiring athletes, weekend warriors, or those unfortunate enough to be on the receiving end of dance floor antics gone wrong!

It is designed to be easily picked up and put down—ideal reading during knee-icing sessions for anyone with a freshly injured knee! After reading the introduction section (Part 1), the athlete chapters (Part 2) can be read chronologically or in any order depending on personal interests in particular sports or individual athletes. These chapters comprise two sections—the nuts and bolts of each athlete's ACL story, and their reflections on their journey through it all. Explanations of technical terms can be found in the glossary at the end. The concluding section (Part 3) can also be read at any stage, and is not to be missed as it contains important practical advice for anyone going through their own ACL injury journey.

The stories in this book will also assist in improving the conversations that need to take place when an ACL injury is sustained. We can all benefit from a greater awareness of what options exist, and what our bodies can achieve with sound management and the hard work required during rehabilitation.

The aim of this book is not to suggest the perfect way to manage, rehabilitate or recover from ACL injury; nor does it intend to be a 'how to' text on ACL rehab and return to sport protocols (these are readily available elsewhere).

Athletes from a variety of sports have been selected, including sports where ACL injuries are not often thought of as common (sailing, cricket), with a cross-section of international approaches to surgical management and/or rehabilitation.

A diverse selection of athletes has been chosen whose stories demonstrate a variety of rehabilitation support and experiences, different graft types, optimal or less-than-optimal outcomes, and conservative versus surgical experiences.

With the focus on the athletes and their stories, the names of all medical and rehabilitation professionals involved have been omitted. The goal is not to point fingers or lay blame where outcomes weren't optimal, but to simply tell each athlete's story in their words, warts and all, so that we can all learn from their experiences—both good and bad.

A NOTE FROM THE AUTHOR

I have always had a love of sport, and an interest in the mechanics of the body, and I have been lucky to combine the two successfully throughout my career. As an Australian-trained Sports and Exercise Physiotherapist I have been fortunate to work alongside some of the world's best athletes and sports medicine teams in Australia and overseas. With such work comes the immense satisfaction of helping athletes achieve their highest of highs—successful Olympic campaigns, World Championships, Grand Finals, and personal bests.

But the biggest sense of fulfilment comes when helping an athlete back from their lowest of lows, as devastating injuries are never far away when you are pushing the limits of physical performance. In my job, that's what it is all about.

From the often dramatic and gut-wrenching buckling of the knee and traumatic 'pop' sensation at the time of the ACL injury, to the usually long and involved rehab required and their time out of sport, no athlete goes through an ACL rupture without having their life upended. But as they say, you need resistance to fly. In my experience the learnings that come from being forced to take time out and change the way you once approached your sport are always immense.

I wasn't always interested in knees and can't say I ever imagined I would create a book solely about ACL injuries. But knees seem to have followed me through my career, particularly from the start of my involvement in winter sports. I worked nomadically through a decade of winter seasons, basing myself in Wanaka, on New Zealand's South Island, during the southern hemisphere winter, and travelling with national teams and athletes (Australia, New Zealand, United States) during the northern winters. In winter sports, ACLs pop like candy. During those years, I assessed and treated more ACL injuries than at any other time in my career.

There are two ACL-injured athletes in particular—Anna Segal and Russ Henshaw, both Australian Olympic Slopestyle skiers, whose scenarios personally and professionally challenged me, and made me rethink what could be possible with the management of ACL injuries. As their physiotherapist I was involved in helping each of them to compete successfully at the 2014 Sochi Winter Olympics with only one intact ACL between them! Their stories are included in the pages that follow; their experiences are what planted the seed for me to write this book.

As well as working in elite sport, I have also consulted in a variety of private-practice settings treating many amateur athletes, weekend warriors, and everyday clients who have sustained ACL injuries. The challenges faced by all who sustain an ACL injury—professional athlete or not—are very often the same.

Physiotherapists are well-positioned to counsel and educate attitudes to ACL injuries, to outline available options (conservative versus surgical), to describe the rehab process, and to motivate and encourage rehab to the end stages. I always tell my athletes and clients that successfully travelling through their ACL journey, although lengthy and often frustrating, will make them the best athlete they've ever been. Over the years I have realised that the stories of others who have travelled this path successfully are louder than any words I or other clinicians could utter. Sharing the ACL journey of a relatable athlete is more powerful and inspiring to a client 'buying-in' to their rehabilitation than any amount of discussion and explanation surrounding the latest ACL research findings or rehabilitation protocols.

I hope that by sharing the ACL journeys of these Australian athletes who have not only rehabbed successfully, but achieved amazing things along the way (with a few tricky moments thrown in), this book will provide an emotional road map on how to work through the injury, to motivate those who have injured their ACL to complete their rehab and not just return to their previous level, but to go beyond, and thus reduce the likelihood of sustaining a recurrent injury.

Jess Cunningham
—June 2022

PART 2

ATHLETES' STORIES

AERIAL SKIING

LYDIA LASSILA

Lydia Lassila is an Olympic champion in aerial skiing who sustained two left-knee ACL ruptures during her career. She underwent reconstructive surgery in Australia for both injuries—utilising an Achilles allograft for the first, and a hamstring graft for the second—and undertook the early stages of her rehabilitations in Australia before progressing to water ramp and on-snow rehabilitations in North America and Europe.

I competed as an aerial skier for Australia over five Winter Olympics. I won gold at Vancouver in 2010, and bronze at Sochi in 2014. As well as winning the medals, I am proud to have pushed the boundaries of my sport and helped bridge the gap between male and female aerial skiers by being the first female to perform a quad-twisting triple somersault—a mission of mine since beginning the sport in 2000. I achieved this while also being a mum to my two sons on tour during my last two Olympic cycles (Sochi and PyeongChang). These days I wear a lot of different hats: retired athlete, mum, wife, business owner, mentor, yoga lover and surfing enthusiast. I love surfing and I love being in the ocean. Like aerial skiing, it allows me to be 100 per cent present whilst filling my void and need for thrill and adrenaline.

It had always been my dream from when I was young to go to the Olympics. Before skiing, I was a national stream gymnast, winning multiple national championships. I showed talent at a young age and was asked to join the elite program, but my parents wouldn't allow it as training was too far from home. It wasn't until I was asked a second time as a 15-year-old, that they finally agreed. But I injured my ankle, and then wrist and as a result wasn't able to make the team for the 1998 Commonwealth Games nor 2000 Olympic Games. I then heard about a program that was turning ex-elite gymnasts into aerial skiers—it was literally a case of one door closing and another door opening. My Olympic goal was still the same, it was just my sport that changed.

I didn't think I could like another sport as much as I loved gymnastics, but I quickly became obsessed with aerial skiing. I was desperate to progress quickly and bypass the beginner stage and go straight to the World Cup level; and that's not far off what happened. Eighteen months after not being able to ski at all I finished eighth at my first Winter Olympics in 2002 in Salt Lake City.

Looking back, it was all a bit nuts to progress that quickly. It was pretty full on. But I was really driven and trained like a work horse. And I was competitive. I had all the makings of what was needed to be a really good athlete. I was as tough as they come. But I was also reckless. At that stage there was no structure within the program, no physios and I overtrained with no objection from my coaches. I jumped with injuries. I did tricks I wasn't ready for. And I guess that behaviour was fed by the fact I was doing well and was progressing, even though my body was getting quite injured.

The injuries started right from the beginning. At the Salt Lake Olympics, I had a torn medial ligament (MCL) in my knee, and I required a shoulder reconstruction soon after. Because I couldn't hold my arm up, I'd started to go crooked off the jump and landing heavily on one leg. As a result, I ended up with a cyst in one of the small joints (L4/5 facet joint) in my lumbar spine. I really wasn't in great shape after those Olympics!

It took me a good few years to start to feel normal again. I kept reinjuring my shoulder each season, and my back was really twisted after all of the punishment I kept putting it through. It was like I needed complete rewiring on my right side. When I think back, I was really quite messed up. At one point I also had a stress fracture in my thoracic spine, bruised ribs, and multiple concussions.

At that stage we didn't have consistent physio for the team. We only had coverage at World Cup events and not at training camps. By that stage, I was already injured and trying to self-manage and cope with ice and Ibuprofen. It wasn't good. My early injury management was all a little too late and reactive. I was constantly pounding myself and wasn't able to get on top of niggles and injuries and improve. It was very difficult.

When I blew my knee the first time, I was on the water ramps in Lake Placid. It was day two of summer training. On my second jump I caught an edge and my knee twisted as I went up the jump. I didn't feel a pop, I just felt a really strong twist on the outside of my knee. I thought I'd just done the lateral ligament. But there was a lot of pain, and it puffed up straight away.

It took a while to diagnose exactly what was wrong. We didn't have a physio with us. I saw local doctors and was sent for an MRI that clearly showed I'd done my ACL. I remember breaking down, thinking my world had come to an end. At that point I was number two in the world. It was only my second year, but I was winning World Cups already and to-ing and fro-ing on the podium with fellow teammate Alisa Camplin. I was doing triples already, and so everything was on track for the Torino Olympics (2006). I'd blown my knee with the Olympics just around the corner. It was July, and the Olympics were in February. It was the worst timing for something like this to happen. It was a disaster.

I flew home and saw our team Doc in Melbourne and got 'booked in' for surgery. Because it was such a short time before the Olympics, it was a question of what were we going to do? My choice was between using a traditional hamstring graft, or an Achilles tendon allograft from a cadaver which was fairly new in 2005. I had a good surgeon, so had confidence in his suggestions and didn't seek any other opinions. The timeframes involved for a hamstring graft meant I would most likely miss the Olympics, and my knee was too unstable to leave it and try conservatively, so we decided to go with the allograft. It would be less invasive and would give me the best chance of recovering in time to try to make it to the Olympics.

After the surgery I progressed really quickly. I had the help of a Victorian Institute of Sport (VIS) trainer and a great physio. It was a pretty intensive rehab to try to get me back. Twice daily at the VIS for bike, leg presses, squats—everything to get me functional again, then daily massage and physio, and constant icing and ice baths. Although we didn't often all sit down together, my team worked well together. There were a lot of unknowns around how hard we could push, but my knee coped, and I made incredible gains in strength and stability.

When it came to getting back on snow, everything was in phases. I moved very quickly through a progression of activities such as box jumps to single leg landings and used my feeling and reaction in my knee as a gauge for when to progress or hold back. However, we were moving really fast. There were a lot of naysayers, but I had to just stay in my lane because it was my knee, my body and my only choice of making it back in time for the Olympics.

I started back skiing at around eight weeks, and returned to the water ramps at three months. I was wearing a custom-made knee brace, but my knee definitely had its flare ups along the way. One of the more memorable episodes happened when I first started back on the water ramps. My coach was from the US, and so hadn't seen me throughout my whole rehab. We first met up again at a camp and he said, 'Look, I have been talking to a lot of people, and they just say this is nuts—that you are back water ramping. Do you mind seeing my specialist in Salt Lake City for a second opinion?' Although I explained I was fine and had been cleared to go, in the end I agreed to see his specialist. They put me on an ACL stress test machine, and it flared up my knee like there was no tomorrow. I was really angry, because everything was tracking well, and then that wrecked my training camp. It really hurt my confidence. My 'team' with whom I had been rehabbing wasn't there, and I was trying to convey everything via Skype. It was really difficult and scary.

Despite the setback I still managed to do enough at that camp to feel comfortable to return to jumping on snow. But I didn't return to triples, as that was now off the cards and too risky. I had to come to grips with the fact that I would just be doing doubles at Torino, as I wasn't going to be able to get the training in, and to take the risk with that extra load on my knee would have been too much.

I was now really particular about how I warmed up. I warmed up for a long time and made sure I did all of my activation exercises before I would get my gear on. I was very, very cautious. If I felt anything that I didn't like I was really quick to call it; which was completely different from that athlete I was before, where I would push through anything. It was a time where I really backed off and wasn't willing to take any unnecessary risks. I was almost timid, which is understandable, because a lot of the time, my knee didn't feel 100 per cent. It was also unchartered territory as we didn't have any reference points of anyone who had come back from ACL surgery in such a short time frame. In the back of my mind, I had a feeling I was doing something that I shouldn't be doing. It was hard.

After the September camp in Utah, I went back into rehab mode until December. I didn't travel with the team to the usual pre-season training camp; I just wanted to wait as long as I could before restarting on snow. I had already qualified for the Olympics because of my great results the year before. So, the plan was to do a couple of the North American World Cups before the Olympics and that would be it.

When I was coming back to jumping on snow, the team was competing in China. This meant I didn't have a coach or a physio. So, I went to our winter training base Apex Mountain Resort in Canada's British Columbia. Training there with me was my old Canadian coach; I asked him for a favour. It seems so strange to talk about this scenario because this would never happen now, but it shows how far our program has come. With me was a Canadian athlete who was also on the comeback. She'd broken her neck at the Mt Buller World Cup in September, and so it was the two of us navigating our injuries and fears together, doing our first jumps together, without any formal support. I was working with a coach who wasn't my coach anymore, and although he looked after me, I really was on my own. He then had to go back home to Whistler for a couple of weeks, so I called up a friend who was also a jumper who lived locally and asked if he could come and stand on the knoll (the flat part next to the jump) and help direct me in the air. The Canadian team also came after Christmas, so I trained with them for a bit too. It just seems so crazy now. There was no physio in the resort, so I'd drive down in the snow to Kelowna, over an hour away, to try to find a therapist. When they'd hear my story, they'd all then provide cautioning opinions.

It took a lot of strength and discipline to deflect the negativity and fear and stay on my path. Despite everything I was going through, I was jumping really well. I was landing everything. I had minimal swelling. I was really controlling everything as much as I could with the resources I had. There was a lot of icing, self-massage, foam rolling, rehab exercises, and taking anti-inflams!

I had started reading a lot of mental training books and listening to visualisation tracks. At that point I didn't have the resources to work with someone in person, but I did practice a lot of visualisation and other mental training techniques. I would keep my jumping numbers to a minimum and then replace the rest with mental imagery training. I felt I was keeping on top of the technical skills by just visualising, rather than actually physically practising. And it was really obvious in the way I was jumping. I made very few mistakes. I had really good landings and take offs. And I was consistent. That was the first time I really understood the power of mental imagery. I was replacing my physical training with visualisation, and I could see the conversion. It was incredible.

Finally, I was reunited with the Australian team in Deer Valley Utah for a World Cup event and had access to consistent physio treatment. It was a double event. I won the first day but decided not to compete on the second day because there was a huge snowstorm. I thought, 'No, I don't need that'. I already had my Olympic qualification, I had a boost of confidence by returning with a win, so I just didn't need the extra risk. I was being cautious and smart.

We went on to Lake Placid for the next World Cup and I trained all through the week and everything was fine. I was managing well. But on contest day, the weather turned foul, so again, I decided not to compete. I did another training camp after that and was again jumping well and managing my knee okay. All up I'd had a good block back on snow. I was landing well. I was hitting my take offs and the tricks I would compete at the Olympics. Most importantly, I was getting back to being comfortable and confident on snow.

We then flew to Torino and instantly my knee just blew up. Nothing caused it. But it was swollen and there was so much crunching and grating going on. It would lock up just walking up the stairs. It would lock up on the bike. My original physio was now with me and the only thing we could put it down to, was the long flight to Europe. My knee was angry and swollen and nothing seemed to help at that stage. That was seven months post-surgery. I don't know how, but I was still able to jump on it. And I was jumping really well. I didn't have any crashes to cause it to flare up. But it remained really angry.

On the day of semi-finals, we'd started jumping, but conditions worsened after a snowstorm. The day's competition was cancelled. I wanted it to go ahead because I was feeling great. I remember turning to my physio and asking if he thought I had two more days in me. And he said, 'Yes, we'll get your knee over the line'.

Once the semi-finals were cancelled there was a traffic jam. Everyone was trying to get out of the snowstorm. My physio and I decided that rather than wait for hours for the bus in my ski boots, we'd walk back to our lodge. It was an uphill walk, but we'd get there quicker. We trudged up in the snow, and my knee was not good. They rescheduled the semi-finals for the next day; by then my knee was in even worse shape. It was getting totally locked up just trying to warm up on the bike. I knew something was brewing.

In the semi-finals my training went well. I landed everything. My first competitive jump was a beautiful jump and had me sitting second, but there's quite a long wait before the second jump. The longer I was waiting the stiffer my knee was getting. Standing around just wasn't good for it. When I got to my second jump, I went a bit big and landed back seat.

I felt it as soon as I hit the ground. It just popped straight away. Gone.

I knew immediately what had happened. I felt a definite 'pop' this time. I was already in a lot of pain with my knee, but this time it really hurt. It hurt a lot. And not just physically. At the time, my teammate Alisa Camplin was also coming back from an ACL injury (after an even shorter timeframe) and incredibly she came away with a bronze medal. She didn't have a great preparation, her training was up and down in the lead-up, yet she managed to put it all together on the day. I was happy for her, but at the same time heartbroken and I asked myself, 'What did I do wrong? Why did this have to happen again?'

I committed to taking a year off. I knew that I needed another reco, and that I was going to use my hamstring as the graft. But there was no way I was going to rush this time. I flew home to Melbourne and saw the same surgeon. I had to have a bone graft first, so they got me in pretty quickly to remove the old graft and plugged up the graft hole with bone from my hip. I had to wait three months for the bone to heal, and then went in for another reco.

The bone graft was really painful. I was shocked by how painful it was. He did a double bundled hamstring graft. There was some talk of using a patella graft, but since I'd had some patella tendinopathy they chose not to do that.

The same trainer and physio were working with me again. But I also started engaging more seriously with a mental coach because I didn't want this to happen to me EVER again. I figured I probably had one chance of another Olympics if I did manage to come back. And I did want to come back, I didn't want to stop. I wanted to make it work, so I was all in this time.

Some interesting discussions were also taking place. I knew that I had to be better managed and have smart people around me to help manage my loads, control the numbers, and just be supportive. Otherwise I was just going to continue to hurt myself if nothing changed.

Finland asked me to jump for them. I had an Italian passport, and so I was seriously considering leaving the Australian system for the European team so I could have access to better facilities, better coaching, and more support staff. I flew to Switzerland and started the process of potentially 'defecting' to Finland. I didn't want to, but I desperately didn't want what happened to me, to happen again to myself or anyone. Discussions became quite serious between all parties, so I put in an ultimatum [to the Australians] requesting full-time physio support in training camps as well as competition, and that I could nominate my own coach. I would only jump for Australia if these support services were in place. We came to an agreement which ended up being better for not just myself, but the whole team and for future generations.

The rehab was pretty similar the second time round, just without the time pressure. I had the support and I engaged a mental training coach. I was pretty traumatised by it all really. Not just physically, but mentally and emotionally as well. I didn't know what I had been doing wrong but could see that the same patterns kept happening to me, and that I needed help. At my first meeting with my mental coach, and after I shared my sob story, he looked me straight in the eye and said, 'You have caused everything that has happened to you'. You can imagine, I really didn't appreciate that comment at the time. He peeled back all of the layers, and in the end, I realised he was right. Everything that had happened I had completely caused, 100 per cent. I wasn't listening to my body by pushing when I should have been pulling back. I did a lot of things right too, but earlier on I probably didn't. Torino was hard because I was so careful and cautious, but it just wasn't meant to be. I had to let go of that one.

I got back on snow in October for my first ski camp in Switzerland. I had a new brace, but it was uncomfortable on the first day. It was rubbing on my hamstring where the graft was taken. I didn't want to wear it but was told that I had to. But by the end of the week I had a Baker's cyst that had formed at the back of my knee. It continued to grow and gave me a lot of trouble. I had to deal with that for the whole season. It was like having a tennis ball at the back of my leg. I was also dealing with constant swelling, constant pain. It was no good. But I was competing well. I was doing just doubles again, but I was really struggling with pain constantly.

At the end of that season I had to get the Baker's cyst removed. The surgeon had to delve down so deep into my joint to get to the root of it, so what I thought would be a two-week recovery period ended up being just as bad as an ACL reconstruction. Aside from the cyst, he found nothing structurally wrong with my knee, so that made it even more frustrating. I could understand if I had bone on bone, or a meniscal tear. But I was being told that I was just always going to have pain in my knee, even though no one could tell me the cause. I just felt there should be a way to get this better and that I shouldn't always be in pain. That's when I started seeking different opinions. I found that my other issues with my back and pelvis were all tied together. My glutes and hip region needed attention in order to support and protect my knee—the previous treatments were always around my knee.

After the Baker's cyst, I never jumped with a brace again. I knew that I was getting irritated by the brace, and that it hadn't been a problem the first time because I hadn't had a hamstring graft. But I could feel the brace digging into my hamstring that was already compromised by being the graft site, and I felt I was compromising it further by strapping it down and inhibiting it; so I just taped my knee whenever I felt I needed to. I really loved the ACL taping with the cross behind the knee. That gave me enough support. I focussed on strength work, preparing my body rather than relying on a brace. And I was fine.

My left knee issues were behind me once I made it to Vancouver for the 2010 Olympics. I did have some right patella pain which was bothering me. I'd never watched my crash in Torino until that point, and my manager sent me through a media clip to approve. On that clip was my crash. I felt like I'd worked for four years to get this out of my head, and two days before my competition someone has shown me the clip that I'd been avoiding for all of those years! It really shook me, but I had enough mental skill at that stage to keep focussing on the future. On top of that, all of my press conference interviews revolved around me blowing out my knee at the last Olympics. Everyone wanted to talk about it. I had to work really hard to deflect and keep my focus. It was constant work.

For some reason I am always a lot more nervous in qualifications than in finals. At Vancouver this rang true again. I didn't perform at my best, but I managed to squeeze through and make it to the finals. The night of the finals was really foggy—you couldn't even see the jumps from the top of the run in. I remember people being a little bit freaked out by the fog, but I felt calm. I had prepared for it. I felt unshakable and was comfortable doing the triple somersaults that I'd wanted to do and planned on doing all through my career. I was on fire and felt I couldn't really put a foot wrong. I was in a great position after landing my first jump, and when I did my final jump, I knew I had it in the bag. It was an amazing final. The quality of the jumping was just incredible. To be able to win, and in that way, was so fulfilling after what I had gone through just to get there.

All of the setbacks and the downs of the knee injuries were worth it, just for that moment. That one sweet moment.

Although many people thought I would, I never called retirement after Vancouver. I didn't want to stop. I loved what I did. I still wanted to do the triple somersaults, and more importantly the quad-twisting triple was a milestone that I desperately wanted to tick. So instead of retiring, I fell pregnant and had my first boy, Kai. I had the intention of coming back as a mum, which just wasn't really done in my sport. It lit a fire in me to prove it was possible. We were trying to navigate new ground, but everyone around me was so supportive. It was worlds away from how I had started in the sport when it had very little structure.

I returned to jumping when Kai was 6 months old and I continued to get strong and fit. My body had changed, but I got back on top of things. I didn't have any issues training on water, but on snow things didn't go so well. I had a lot of back and pelvis issues in the 2012 season. Trying to compete for the whole season with bulging discs in my back was excruciating. We didn't pick up early enough that my pelvis was still a little bit unstable after childbirth, even though I felt very strong. My stabilising muscles withered down to zero throughout the season with all of the pain. I wasn't in a good place at all.

Training and travelling with Kai was tough. We managed, but I had to be very strong. I even cut my hair short to help me feel stronger. With so many people doubting my return post Kai, my back injury, my ability to do triple somersaults with four twists, it fuelled my ambition to defend my title at Sochi. I was really on a mission.

Once back in Australia, I was able to get my back and stabilising muscles on track again. I prepared for Sochi really well, but we had a lot of bad weather leading in to the Games which made it difficult to get much practice in for the triple-twisting quad. It wasn't until I was at Sochi that I managed to do it in training, just a couple of days before the Games. Not the place you usually try new tricks!

**During the training session right before the competition at Sochi, I came up short and landed on the knoll. I hyperextended my left knee and heard this big 'crack'. I immediately thought it was all over. I couldn't put weight on it, and when I'd fully extend, it would give me this incredible amount of pain. I missed most of the training because I was getting assessed and strapped by our doc and physio. I just kept thinking, 'Not now, not now'. It turned out I'd damaged my meniscus, but my ACL was okay. They strapped my knee so I couldn't fully extend it, and if I kept it warm the pain was reduced somewhat. But that was difficult to do on a snowy hillside throughout the entire six-hour competition format. If it cooled down too much, the pain would come straight back.

Despite it all, I jumped well and made it through to the super-final round where four competitors did a final jump to decide the medals. I went for the quad-twisting triple. It was only my third time doing the jump on snow. I wanted it all. I wanted to defend my Olympic title and win, and I wanted to do that trick. I went for it but didn't land cleanly and came away with the bronze medal. Even though I didn't win, I certainly won a spot in history by being the first woman to do that trick and I've come to appreciate my Olympic medals more over time. Olympic medals are not easy to come by, whatever the colour.

I fell pregnant again after Sochi. This time I thought it would be time to retire. But I still felt the pull of the sport. I loved jumping and being an athlete—I didn't want to stop, so I didn't. I had a completely different mindset this time though. It wasn't for an Olympic medal. I didn't want to push the boundaries anymore. I just wanted to enjoy my final moments as an athlete, do good quality jumping and transition out of sport in my own way and basically say goodbye to that life and the people and places in it.

I restarted my training two years out from PyeongChang. Training and competing with two small children was definitely a juggle. I look back now and wonder, 'What was I thinking?'. But I was still winning World Cups, was very competitive and I was having fun.

At PyeongChang my training went really well. I didn't fall once, until in qualifications, where I didn't land either of my jumps. And that was it.

It was over, finished. I was shattered not to make the final. But I just didn't have the same toughness I'd had four years earlier. I wasn't plagued by knee issues or any other injuries. But it just wasn't my night and I couldn't seem to find my focus when I needed it. It wasn't the way I was hoping to end my career. But I was finally ready to retire.

I am still bothered today by something in the back of my ACL knee, and I have some ongoing patella tendonitis in my right knee. But I can still do everything I'd like to do in my life. Mostly because I have learned how to manage and look after myself through yoga and stability exercises.

REFLECTIONS

Looking back, my ACL experiences definitely weren't what I expected. They were rocky. They were like my whole career, which has been filled with constant ups and downs.

I was pretty disheartened when I was told I'd done my ACL the first time. I had big plans for Torino—I was going to win! I was doing triple somersaults and really coming on strong. It felt like everything came crashing down, and I kept thinking, 'Why has this happened to me?'. I'd trained so hard, whereas other people who didn't never seemed to get injured. It wasn't until I started working with my mental coach during my second ACL rehab that I realised I had caused everything that happened to me. I did overtrain. I did push too hard. I hadn't yet learned how to periodise and taper, or to pace myself. The mental training was an intensive learning block that really helped me to accept what had happened, and to accept that everything that happened was a sequence of behaviours and thought processes that I had created which led to my ACL injuries. Once I understood that, I could be more mindful of all of my behaviours moving forward.

I learned how to process and filter out what was going to be useful to me and throw out what wasn't. I learned how to observe and understand how I reacted in situations where I felt threatened or a loss of confidence. That was so important in coming back for my next Olympic campaign. Everyone knew what happened to me in Torino, and every journalist bought it up, along with the fact that I wanted to do triple somersaults and that I was coming back from a double knee reco. It was just constant. Everyone was talking about it all. And even my family too—asking if I really needed to be doing this anymore—'Don't you think you've had enough?' The mental side was crucial. It really helped me to focus.

My mental coach was also really critical in helping me reframe my previous behaviours. Particularly me saying and thinking, 'These things always happen to me and I'm always injured', to instead, 'Look I've had some injuries in the past, but that doesn't mean it's going to happen to me again. My past doesn't equal my future'. That was really important for me in training, in rehab, in everything. I was always projecting to the stronger recovered Lydia that I wanted to be—the Lydia who was doing triples, and the Lydia who won a gold medal.

I had great support through the VIS, but aerial skiing means you are overseas for much of the year. Coming back from an ACL you need the consistency of physio and strength and conditioning work through the whole process. For me it was very stop-start when I went overseas, and it was really hard for me to know what to do. If there was a flare up, what do I do? If I was feeling a bit of pain here, what was the cause of it? Now things are different, and winter athletes don't get sent away without that kind of support especially when they are intensively rehabbing. For me, that was a big hole in my preparation. If I'd had someone there consistently to help me with strength and conditioning, I wouldn't have been in such a reactive kind of state all the time. I would have been able to manage my body a lot better.

My knee issues definitely made me a smarter athlete. I wasn't going to make the same mistakes again. As well as making me invest in the mental side of things, I also started my business *BODYICE* too because I couldn't find icepacks that wouldn't slip all over the place! In hindsight it was the best thing that could have happened to me. It really forced me to have perspective, and take time away from the sport and I developed other interests, and a business. That business then gave me the flexibility and financial means to train wherever I wanted, to have whoever I wanted as a mental coach, and get all of the extra things and equipment I needed. It continues to expand and still supports me to this day. My knee experiences, although unpleasant at the time, completely changed me for the better.

My injuries (not just my knees) also taught me to seek out second opinions. If there was no structural damage, then why was I in so much pain? I always pushed to find out why, and if my team didn't have the answers, then I would seek answers elsewhere. Through that process I found yoga, and Pilates. If I hadn't found my Pilates guy, they were going to singe a nerve in my back. If I hadn't found my mental coach, I wouldn't have made it to Vancouver. I wouldn't have returned to the level I got to without these people, no way. Not to the stage where I was pushing the boundaries and doing tricks women hadn't done before after everything that I'd gone through. When I had bulging discs in my back, if I hadn't found my yoga guy, I wouldn't have made it to the next two Olympics. Being able to understand and manage my body, and my mind, and having the team that could help me do that gave me an extra three Olympics.

Taking a non-surgical approach was definitely on my mind. I had people close to me who were skiing successfully without an ACL. Swiss aerials skier Evelyne Leu won the 2006 Olympics without an ACL, and my husband Lauri, competed in mogul skiing without an ACL. But my joint just wasn't stable enough, so it was never really an option for me. My husband's knee is quite stiff so he could do it, but I am hypermobile, and my knee was just loose. It all depends on your anatomy. It isn't an option for everyone. If it's functional and stable then great, but if not it's just not an option.

It is hard to say when in my menstrual cycle my ACL injuries occurred. As an athlete I've always used a Mirena IUD. My periods were very light before that and never a big deal for me performance-wise, so my main reason for the Mirena was contraception rather than performance. It was just presented to me as a better option than having to remember to take the pill every day. I had a really positive experience with it and never had any side effects, so it worked well for me. Interestingly I remember that the Chinese team never jumped when they had their period, they were always on the sidelines. I don't know if that was for performance or cultural reasons. I found that quite odd at first but am more curious about it now knowing that menstrual cycle hormone changes can be associated with ACL injury.

If I could give advice to my former self, it would be don't train harder, but train smarter—to understand that for my body to carry me through 17 years of sport, I've got to look after it in order for it to look after me. And to seek help earlier. But I feel that within my power and with the resources I had, I did everything I could. That's what you have to accept. But do I know better now? Of course I do. Because I went to the school of hard knocks and I learned what I was doing was reckless and wrong in the beginning, which led to other injuries that compromised my body and my career. But you don't know what you don't know. Could I have avoided a lot of situations had I been better managed from the beginning? Definitely.

To those who have injured their ACL, a big part of coming back successfully is the emotional and mental recovery. You need a positive mindset surrounding your recovery and your rehab, because there are going to be days when you're up, and days when you're down. If you are returning to sport, in particular a sport that is quite risky and high impact, you need to reframe what has happened to you and be able to confidently project from that injury and not dwell on past trauma. I think the mental and emotional component is equally as important as medical support.

AMERICAN FOOTBALL

ADAM GOTSIS

Adam Gotsis is an American National Football League (NFL) player who has sustained two ACL injuries, both to his left knee. He underwent surgery for each in the USA, using a hamstring graft initially, and a quadriceps graft after his recurrence. His rehabilitations were both completed in America.

I was born and raised in Melbourne. At 19 I moved to the United States on a college scholarship to play American football for Georgia Tech. At the end of my senior year in 2016, I became the highest-ever Australian drafted in the 2016 NFL draft, at pick 63 for the Denver Broncos. I spent the next four years with the Broncos, before becoming a free agent and being signed by the Jacksonville Jaguars in 2020. I am still with the Jaguars.

Sport has been my life and I've loved it right from the start. At six I started playing Australian football with AFL Auskick, before getting into cricket, basketball, tennis—any sport I could get my hands on. At 15 I was selected to play AFL with the Oakleigh Chargers in the NAB league, but it didn't really work out how I imagined. That pushed my AFL dream away, as I realised it wasn't going to be where I could make a career.

I was a big guy, but I wasn't seven feet tall, so I knew basketball was out of the equation too. I had more of a rugby player's build, so thought I'd jump into that. But I didn't even get the chance as my Mum found a flier for an American football team tryout. 'You should try this!' she said. So, I went.

There was no AFL Auskick version of building things up slowly. Under 14s to under 19s was all one age group. I remember seeing how big everyone was and I was thinking: 'I'm not getting out of the car. I'm not going'. My brother ended up coming with me for moral support, but he actually excelled at the sport himself! Once I got going, I loved it, absolutely loved it. I felt like I belonged more than ever and that it was my sport.

I never really had any serious injuries when I was younger. Aside from a few ankle sprains, my one real injury was at 17 when I broke my collarbone playing American football. I didn't need surgery, it just healed. I was really healthy throughout my whole college career with just a few muscle strains here and there, and a slight meniscus injury in my freshman year, but never anything that needed surgery or caused me to miss serious game time.

It was halfway through my senior season in college when I tore my left ACL. I was in the best shape of my life and felt invincible after having done so much hard training through the four-year grind of college. I was at my peak. But unfortunately, my season got cut short. On Halloween of all days!

It was the first play of the game. My opponent was trying to block me, and we were wrestling and pushing each other. I went to push off, and then, suddenly, I was down on the ground. I didn't feel a pop or anything like that in my knee. It felt like I got tripped, but there was no contact. The trainers came out and I remember saying it felt like I needed to crack my knee like a knuckle, you know, to feel that click and relief. I didn't think I was seriously hurt, there wasn't much pain or swelling. It just felt weird.

I was able to walk off the field and the doctor assessed my knee. I've got pretty big legs, so it's hard to grab my legs and get a good feel of my ligaments, especially on the sidelines when you're sitting on a bench. But he said it felt okay as I didn't have any signs or symptoms of a serious injury and asked to see if I could run down the sidelines. I took off jogging and ran for about a dozen steps, before the whole knee gave way. My whole leg just collapsed inwards; it felt like the outside of my foot touched the outside of my knee. I felt it pop that time, and that's when I knew it was something serious. I then went inside the locker room with the doctor and he looked at it again, and he was 99 per cent sure it was my ACL, but said we'd get an MRI to be certain.

The next day my knee was pretty sore, although the swelling didn't get too crazy. Two days later the MRI showed my ACL was torn. It was all pretty disappointing.

I did 10 days of prehab trying to get my quads firing before having surgery. I felt extremely comfortable and had a good relationship with our team surgeon. I'd seen guys progress well with him, including a friend who had torn his ACL the year before and ended up getting drafted. When we talked about the best type of graft to use, he wasn't a big fan of cadavers because he felt your cells respond better to having your own materials in your body. And with patella tendon, he mentioned tendonitis and arthritis can be an issue. He felt my quad tendon was so thick he could take a graft and I wouldn't lose much integrity, so that's what we went with.

Unfortunately, I ended up with an infection at the graft site. On day five post-surgery, I voiced concern as it was red and raised around the stitches, but the college docs didn't seem too worried. When I saw my surgeon around two weeks later, he agreed it looked infected—most likely from the college training room environment with so many athletes coming and going, and the tables and icing compression sleeves not often being cleaned or changed. I ended up having my whole knee cleaned out. I stayed in hospital for a week with a PICC line in my arm and on antibiotics. Once home, I had to keep the line in for another four weeks and inject a bunch of medications through it every eight hours. It had to be wrapped every time I had a shower. It was crazy. Everything was put on hold for a month because with a PICC line in you can't sweat or really do much, as if anything gets into that line it's going straight into your heart and can lead to bigger complications. I didn't need any of those.

I was able to start rehabbing in early January once I got the PICC line out. I finally felt I was on track without any roadblocks or hiccups in the way. With the NFL Scouting Combine in late February, I had some time to get myself into decent shape. I knew I wouldn't be able to run at the Combine, but they have other tests like bench press, so I was keen to train for that. I'd go in and rehab in the morning, then hit the weights room for strength and upper body lifting. I wanted to get my knee in the best condition I could because I knew it was going to get tugged and pulled on by a lot of people during the evaluations—all 32 teams are at the Combine with all their medical staff.

The Combine week was pretty intense. There were six rooms, each with around six teams in each, and a table in the middle. You'd walk in and sit at the table while a doctor from each team would come up and do all of their tests on you. Then you'd go to the next room and go through the same evaluations again. It was a weird experience. But if a team's going to invest in you, they need to see exactly what they're about to invest in. I only heard good things about my body in response from the doctors there. I felt pretty good at that point.

I ended up getting drafted to the Broncos and transferred to Denver in May. I thought it would be a smooth transition. But Georgia Tech's timeline for a return from ACL was a bit longer than the Broncos', and I got stuck between the two different protocols. I could tell pretty quickly that things weren't on the same page. I was doing some running before I left for the Broncos, but once I got there, they backed me off to go back to focus on strengthening exercises rather than movement. Once I started doing field work with the athletic training staff, I really only ran for a week or so. Then it was doing individual drills with my position coach, things like footwork, change of direction, and agility bag work for a week before I was given a knee brace and sent out to practise with the team.

I was cleared to play at the end of July—around eight months after the surgery. Because the infection delayed me starting my rehab until January, despite my ACL surgery being in November, it was really more like seven months. I didn't think I was ready to be back in that time, but as I was being pressured by training staff and coaches, I felt that I didn't have an option.

Not surprisingly my first season didn't go that great. I didn't have any confidence in my knee. I went from not playing football, to playing 35 plays every pre-season game—which is a lot, especially coming off an injury. It felt like my knee never really got to heal, and then I was putting all of this pounding and wear and tear on it. Especially in the position I play (defensive tackle) where you're going up against guys that are 130kg to 140kg, and sometimes it's two guys on one. You've really got to have a strong base and to make sure that you have the same conditioning and strength you had previously to be able to perform at that high level.

I was trying to play at 100 per cent, but I felt like I was only at 80 per cent. It just wasn't working. I couldn't even run at times. Often after games I would be hobbling around. But I'd do what I could to get it ready for the next week and go out there and do it all again. That's was my mentality. It was pretty bad. And at the end of the season, I couldn't even squat 60kg. My left hip and ankle also felt all locked up, which couldn't have been helping my knee.

After the season I needed a lot of work. However, I didn't feel the exercises I was given from the training staff were enough to get me back to playing well. So, in the off-season I went back to Georgia Tech for a few months of rehab with my original support team. It got me back to feeling like I was an athlete again. I also got into yoga and stretching a lot, and that really helped.

I came back to the Broncos feeling really healthy. It was like I was back to myself with running. I felt close to 90 per cent. Through the next two years (2017, 2018), I stayed pretty healthy, even though I was still playing in a custom-made ACL brace underneath my pads for extra support. It never felt great playing with the brace, but I just had to convince myself that this was just a part of my uniform.

My knee never quite got back to feeling 100 per cent. Halfway through the 2018 season I felt a bit of a shift in my left knee. I had an MRI and the medical team said I'd stretched the ACL a bit and there was a bit of meniscal wear and tear, but nothing that required surgery. I continued playing out the season, but I was in a bit of pain, on pain killers and anti-inflammatories before every game. When I could no longer take anti-inflammatories as they were messing with my stomach, I took turmeric and tried to find other natural remedies to help me through. On top of the treatment and rehab I was doing with the Broncos, I also took it upon myself to get a lot of work done outside the facility—chiropractic, massage, and acupuncture, all of which I feel really helped.

At the end of the season, I met with the team docs for my exit physical. I asked if there was anything more we could do for my knee, perhaps stem cells or PRP injections. They felt the risks outweighed the rewards, which I didn't agree with completely but with them being my employer I took their advice and didn't pursue anything. But during the 2019 offseason workouts with the team, it got to the point where I felt I couldn't make it through a season with my knee in its condition. I ended up getting PRP injections into the joint and graft in June. That delayed decision only left me with one month before training camp started, rather than the three to four months to recover, which annoyed me. But I got through training camp, and my knee was feeling better for the most part. A lot of the pain and inflammation went down, but I still wasn't above 90 percent.

By late 2019 I ended up tearing it again in a game. It was the third play of the game and I tried to make a move, but my foot got stuck in the ground and I felt my knee shift again. I didn't feel it completely give way—it was more of a tug. I ended up playing the rest of the game, hoping it was just a bit of a freak thing and that I'd be okay. I talked to the docs after the game and they said to come in the next day to have a look at it.

At this point I didn't have the best trust in the medical and training staff, so I asked for a second opinion. You're allowed to do that for any injury. I sent the MRI to a specialist in Vail who was recommended by my agent, along with the MRI I'd had in 2018 when I first felt that shift in my knee. He told me I'd probably been playing on a torn ACL for the last year and a half. He also told me I had a grade 4 medial meniscus tear, some lateral meniscus damage, as well as a cyst in my femur where the top screw was. The team hadn't mentioned any of this. They only described everything very vaguely. I felt like I hadn't been told the full story for the last 18 months.

When I went to see the new surgeon, he was pretty straight forward with everything. One option was to have two surgeries—a bone graft and clean out around the cyst, with three to four months to let the bone heal, before redoing the ACL. But the surgeon was confident he could do everything in one go. He was able to work around the cyst and drain it (it's still in there but a lot smaller), and used a patella graft from my other (right) knee thinking it would be better to have the bone-to-bone attachment considering everything else that was going on in my knee. The surgery lasted about seven hours, and he told me he broke three saw tips trying to get the graft! It was pretty brutal. The next week I was pretty sore!

After the surgery there were only a handful of games left in the season, so I just focussed on my rehab. I wasn't really involved with the team any more other than coming in for rehab each day. My contract was expiring, so I had to figure out where I would finish my rehab. I ended up at a private facility in Golden, Colorado where they had experience working with professional athletes. It was like a fresh start. Instantly I felt totally welcome. They progressed me through all of the stuff I thought I would be doing the first time around, but didn't— field work, lots of change of direction, drills with a trainer and pads, and so much more single leg strength work. They gave me a lot of attention for the few months I was with them. Their whole mentality was to get me back to being the best and most functional player I could be.

They did just that. My knee now feels more like 95 per cent. And it isn't swollen at all. It occasionally gets a little bit of an ache, but it's really not noticeable. I can now go walking and for a run without thinking about it or feeling like it might buckle or give way, compared to the previous four years where if I didn't have a knee brace on, I don't think I could have run even 50 metres. It's like I've been with a mechanic getting a tune up, and now here I am with a whole new knee. I am looking forward to a new chapter with the Jacksonville Jaguars.

REFLECTIONS

My experience with ACL injury has definitely been a journey—an awesome one. Going through some tough times over the past few years has set me up for not only a good comeback and return to NFL, but for a better life in the long run.

When I was told I'd done my ACL in college, there were a lot of emotions. I knew it was the end of my season, and I thought I was going to miss out on the NFL Combine. But I was also team captain that year, and initially I didn't even care about myself. I was just so disappointed I couldn't be there on the field for the guys to finish out the season. That was probably the hardest part. I still tried to maintain the captain's role and be there as a leader at practice and games, but it hurt to be around just watching it all.

Once I accepted the injury had happened and I couldn't change it, I shifted my mindset to being super-motivated. I figured I would do everything the doctors said and maintain a positive attitude as I still had my chance to go to the NFL. I was going to come back from it. I was going to get drafted to a team somewhere. The infection was a bit of a setback, but once I got into the rehab it felt like I was on my way. I had my family visit from Australia, and I had a tonne of support from the people around me at Georgia Tech—teammates, their families, and the school itself, they all showed me a lot of love.

Once I transitioned to the Broncos it was hard to keep my positive attitude going. With my last two months of rehab not what I thought it should be, it felt like they were pushing me in a way I wasn't ready to be pushed; but I didn't know how to tell them that. It felt like I had no one in my corner. I became miserable and started to have doubts. I didn't have a great relationship with my agent at that point, I'd lost confidence in the training staff, and it didn't feel like I had the support of the coaching staff, or that the team was on my side because of that. It was more like: 'Oh, he can't even play. He can't even run'. It felt like there was a lot of negative energy towards me which definitely didn't help.

I felt alone. It was a dark time. I didn't have anyone else there to reach out to, or who reached out to me other than family. I did have some talks with the team's sports psychologist but didn't wish to pursue that line as I didn't feel like sharing information with them. I tried to be as positive as I could, but it was really hard to hang in there. In the end I didn't even feel comfortable going into the facility. I didn't feel like I belonged in that place. There was so much negativity, anxiety and stress. It was really hard to feel like that and still turn up and show your face. It was definitely a rough couple of years after that first ACL. Mentally it took more of a toll on me than physically.

No one from my inner circle reached out to ask if I was okay, as I hid my emotions from them well. My sisters came to visit from Australia, but I couldn't talk to them because I didn't want them to see me hurting and struggling. I also felt I couldn't reach out to my old college teammates and say, 'Hey, I'm not doing that great', because they all wanted to be in my position—me having been drafted and playing NFL. It was tough. Even to my friends, everyone thought I was happy and that everything was going so well, but I wasn't happy at all. It was mentally the worst time of my life. I isolated myself a lot with my emotions and it messed with my mind so much. I lost myself.

Once I was injured again, it was almost a relief—I could get my issues sorted. My goal for the second rehab was just to get as healthy as I could, and not to worry about landing on a team. I felt if I could stay focussed on the rehab, the rest would take care of itself. I tried to think of it as if I'd been given a second chance to go through it all again, but to do it right this time. I was also hoping to get a fresh start with a new team where no one knew of my past.

During my rehab I was approached by a guy who ran a foundation around men's mental health. He thought I could be a good bridge for Australian audiences at some of his seminars. Through talking to him and opening up about my experiences, I was in tears at points. But it helped me understand what had been going on and how to categorise it. Once I could do that, I was able to move away and detach myself from it. Then I was able to open up to my family more, and my partner, and explain to them where I was at. It was such a relief no longer having to hold all the pressure in, because at the root of it all I didn't want to disappoint my family. I didn't want to let them down or show them I was weak and couldn't do it. Whether that was ego, or the competitor in me, I don't know.

Now I have a great support group around me and feel like I'm me again as a person. I'm back to feeling good about myself and what is around me. I carry myself better. I don't feel like I'm an isolated, introverted person. I'm back to seeing the positives in life, and I have love to share with the world again. It's like a second birth. I'm looking to the future and living and building and growing, rather than just sheltering from everything. I'm opening up and becoming a human again. I'm communicating with my sisters, brother and parents much more—and they notice it. I can tell our relationships have grown so much and have become so much stronger, because I feel better about myself. Everything is as good as it can be again.

If I had the same experience now, I would easily be able to stand up for myself and express how I am really feeling. When I first did my ACL, I was only 23 and didn't know how to handle the ups and downs of serious injury, but also having been through it all, I've seen I'm not the only one who's had this experience. And that definitely puts me in a position where I now feel confident advocating for men's mental health awareness.

I've learned a lot of patience with myself and my body over the years. Mentally I realised the importance of having good support and positive energy around me. If your head space isn't there you can do so much damage to yourself, and once that happens, your body is next to go no matter how hard you try.

Years of receiving a lot of body work—massage, acupuncture, and stretch—also really allowed me to get in tune with my body and understand how it works. I learned to listen to my body, understand what it was telling me, and then act accordingly, rather than just pushing as hard as I could all the time. I feel I'd be a great physiotherapist at this point!

I'm at the stage now where I've found a recipe that works for me. It's just maintaining that now—whether it's the training, nutrition, or mental health side. I feel I now have my fingers wrapped around it all, compared to my first injury when I was just going off everyone else's advice. But what works for me might not work for the next person, and that's the thing about an injury—everyone's body is different. We all heal differently.

I've had two significant injuries to my knee, and it's got to be an ongoing point of focus with the preventative stuff. Just keeping that going is huge: working on the little things and developing routines and staying true to them. I definitely take a lot more measures than someone who hasn't injured their knee. But that's just part of my preparation now. I'll arrive at the stadium early, jump in the hot tub, stretch, roll out, and do some balance work to get my muscles switched on and activated before a game. The preparation is just as important as the play.

I've heard of players playing without ACLs before, but our window is so short in NFL (it's called 'Not For Long' for a reason—there are not a lot of 30-year-olds playing!). There's not much choice other than to get the surgery, recover, and get back as soon as you can. We're also a lot bigger than your average guy. I'm not so sure a player weighing 130-140kg would go that well not having ligament support there.

I think the conversation needs to shift to more of a preventative focus rather than reactive. I've noticed a change in that in the last couple of years in the NFL. The new strength and conditioning coaches have been doing a lot more preventative stuff. But I think there still needs to be a bigger focus on it, not only at the pro level but with young athletes as well. There are so many young kids out there tearing their ACLs, and many of these could be prevented just with better training.

If I could go back in time, I'd get on top of the body work before the injury got to a point where it was on top of me. That's something I didn't do very well the first time around. I didn't have the financial resources to invest in myself. I wasn't aware of the work needed. I was getting massage at Georgia Tech, but once I got to the Broncos I figured they would see that I was doing all of the rehab, lifting all of the weights, and practising as hard as I could, but I wasn't doing anything for recovery other than hot/cold tubs. I didn't know how important that part would be.

I would also tell my former self to keep a confident and positive attitude. To not let negative people and energy get inside my headspace; don't let the environment or the people around you dictate who you are as a person. Stay true to yourself.

Advice to others would be to stay positive and consistent. Understand that yes, you're injured, but you're going to come back and you can come back better than you were. It's not the end of the world. Surround yourself with good people. And keep that circle small, made up of people who genuinely care about you as a person, not just as an athlete.

For the injury itself, do the little things. Don't skip over them. And make sure you're doing your recovery because you're pushing your body, and it's been through a traumatic accident. When your body's telling you it's sore, understand it. Recover, stretch, do what you have to do to get it back to being ready. Understand that you are the one who is responsible for your body.

It's a long road, and you're going to run into speed bumps, but understand they are just speed bumps. They're not blockages. They're not stop signs.

When the going gets really tough, you're going to find out about yourself and who you really are. When the doubt creeps in: 'Can I do this?', that's where your support system comes in. It's going to push you through that and help you to find a way to get past it.

Ultimately, I've come to learn that injuries happen. When adversity strikes you've got to keep working, put your head down, trust your body, and sometimes just work smarter and not always harder. What you put in is what you get out mentally and physically. There's hardship but there's a light at the end of the tunnel.

Even if you don't return to play, you learn a lot about yourself through the process. You grow as an individual. If you can stay on that path, I think it will be really beneficial in the long run.

FOOTBALL (SOCCER)

LYDIA WILLIAMS

Lydia is an Australian soccer player who has sustained two ACL injuries in her career - both to her left knee. Her reconstructive surgeries were conducted in Australia utilising a hamstring graft for the first, and patella graft for the second. She completed the early stages of her first rehabilitation in Australia, before returning to Sweden for the end stages, and her second rehabilitation was conducted solely in Australia.

I am the goalkeeper for the Matildas, Australia's women's football (soccer) team. I've been playing with the national team for more than 15 years, which has taken me to four FIFA World Cups, two Olympics, and five Asian Cups. I also currently play for Arsenal in the UK's Women's Super League (WSL). Previously I played in Australia's W League with Canberra United and Melbourne City, as well as in the USA in the National Women's Soccer League (NWSL) with Western New York (formerly Buffalo), Chicago, Washington, Houston, and Seattle. In my early years I also played for Pitea in the Swedish Damallsvenskan League. My soccer skills were better than my Swedish that's for sure!

I grew up in Kalgoorlie in Western Australia and as most country kids do, played sport on weekends—soccer, basketball and little athletics. I also played Australian rules football, learning to kick and catch a footy in the desert when we'd go out to Indigenous communities. When I was 11, we moved to Canberra. With no footy or real athletics at the time, I basically got stuck playing basketball and soccer, and futsal (a form of indoor soccer). At around 14 I realised I needed to focus on soccer if I wanted to be serious about playing.

I have been a goalkeeper since we moved to Canberra. I arrived late into registration, and goalkeeper was the only position left in Division 1. Not wanting to drop divisions, I accepted the spot, thinking we would rotate, as that's what we had done in WA. But I soon realised that wasn't to be the case, and was stuck with the position! It has worked out quite well for me!

Before my knee, injuries had been kind to me. My only real issue was a broken scaphoid that required surgery in 2008. I was already playing for the national team, and there was no time between tours for me to have surgery straight away. So, I continued to play with a wrist brace and broken scaphoid for another six months, until there was an opportunity to get it fixed.

I did my knee during my first season playing in Sweden in 2012. It was only my second game. I was 24 years old. I remember a ball got played over the top and I was in the wrong position. I came sprinting out for it, but as I was running, I knew I wasn't going to get there. I stopped and planted on my left to push off to my right, and I just felt this 'pop' sensation. Unfortunately, the other team scored. I got up, and straight away knew something wasn't right. I could feel something at the back of my knee and thought maybe I'd pulled my hamstring. I tried to do a few hammy stretches, but it didn't feel stable.

The physio came out and said not to worry. But a few minutes later I tried to turn and side-shuffle down the sideline in my goal and it just felt completely unstable and I went down. They took me off. I tried to walk, but my knee started swelling and feeling really tight. I was like, 'Oh I really hope this isn't what I think it is!'. I remember sitting in the changerooms and straight away calling my mum. I knew something was wrong and that I had to get it scanned and assessed.

That night I hobbled home from the game. I wasn't really putting any pressure on my leg. I saw the physio again the next morning who agreed it needed to be scanned. The scan happened the next day, but they couldn't really tell what was going on. I said, 'What do you mean you can't tell what's going on?!'. But it was obviously an old MRI machine. Everything was sent back to the national team, and they thought it didn't look good, but agreed I needed it rescanned. When I sent through the second lot of images, they could finally confirm I'd done my ACL.

At that time there were quite a few ACLs happening in our national team. I think there were six or seven girls who'd had a recent ACL injury, so I knew, from talking to them, what their experiences were like and how they felt it happen. But I was one of the first to do my ACL in the Swedish team I was playing with. It was a small town and the physio was relatively new so hadn't perhaps seen that many ACL injuries. It didn't really swell that much—there was more pain than swelling—and I think because of that they weren't quick at recognising the signs. I also think that for everyone's sake they didn't want it to be true.

The Swedish club was willing to take care of the surgery, but the national team wanted me to come home right away to have my ACL repaired in Australia. It was a bit of back and forth for a couple of days trying to figure out the best plan. I was just happy to follow recommendations. I also had a bit of meniscus that had flipped the wrong way which was causing me a lot of pain. I didn't think I would last a 30-hour flight and transfers with the kind of pain I was in, so I went under for an arthroscope in Sweden. There was no pain when I woke up, and I was able to fly back to Australia after around five days. I went on blood thinners and had to inject myself before and during flights to make sure there was no blood-clotting.

I first went home to Canberra, and then flew to Adelaide to see our team doctor. I went through the ACL surgery process there at around three weeks post-injury. I stayed in Adelaide for around a week post-surgery, before returning to Canberra.

I had a hamstring graft. There was some discussion about the different types of grafts, but the surgeon had done all of our national team players ACLs and they all had hamstring grafts. I think that was kind of the standard practice at that point in time.

We had a 12-month window, dictated by the medical team. It took me out for the rest of the Swedish season, which was fine with me. There was no pressure to return to playing too quickly.

After the surgery, I fought hard to be able to complete my rehab back in Sweden. I knew that mentally if I was in Australia it would be a struggle, because at that time we didn't have a full-time program and there weren't any camps or teams I could be around. Although it took a bit of convincing from both sides to put together a plan we were all happy with, it was decided I would do the initial three months in Australia until I got to running, then I'd fly to Sweden and finish everything there. I was probably thought to be a little rebellious for wanting to do that, but I knew there was no way I could get through in a good mental state if I just stayed at home.

As a result, I really did have quite the international and domestic ACL experience! The conversations all took place between our Australian physio and doctor and the Swedish club's physio, trainer and doctor. Initially I was also lucky to work with an old national team physio based in Canberra who had seen me growing up through the Canberra system before I made national teams. He guided me to the point where the national team was comfortable that I could run, hop, land and jump.

A main focus in that period was building bulk and strength in my quads. I take a bit longer than some to build muscle, but as we weren't time-pressured, and it wasn't like I was going to be forced into anything too difficult in Sweden, the approach was simply: 'Here's our plan, reach these points, make sure you have these things ticked off'. I was lucky to have good support around me.

The only minor setback was at around the two-month mark. I forgot about my hamstring graft and bent over. It literally felt like I'd been shot in the back of the leg. It subsided relatively quickly, and we didn't get it scanned, but since then my hamstring was a bit tricky to fully regain its strength.

Once I returned to Sweden, I worked with their physio. Before training we'd either do running drills, or some passing, and then when the team came out, I'd do gym and more rehab stuff. As soon as I could do more, I would work into goalkeeper handling and light movements and then we'd do more running and jumping. It was all very tailored to my needs. I was lucky to have an American teammate who had also rehabbed her ACL, so she gave me a lot of support and ran me through some stuff she'd done in the US. It was nice to have her there.

I returned to playing competition at around 11 and a half months. I eased in gradually starting at 30 minutes playing time. I didn't wear a brace, and I didn't tape either. I just relied on my muscles. I felt 100 per cent with regards to my knee, but I didn't feel my normal self, performance-wise. It probably took another year for me to restore full confidence in my playing ability. That took me into 2013-14.

I was away from the national team for much of that time. We also had a new coach in while I was rehabbing. When I returned there were differences in how we prepared for training. We now had a prehab program to follow, leading into camps and training sessions. And ever since, that process has stuck with me—I do the exercises before every training and game.

After that everything was going great. I stayed in Australia and won the League with Canberra. I didn't know if I wanted to play overseas again, as I was enjoying playing and being at home. But I got a phone call from Buffalo in the US asking, 'Would you come over? You've got American citizenship. We'd love to have you over here.' Their goalkeeper had just done her ACL in preseason. I had to make a decision within a few weeks and ended up accepting the offer and packing my bags. At that point the US League was the next up-and-coming 'big thing', and it was exciting to be one of the first Australians to be playing there. I think there were only five of us at that point. I arrived and completed whatever was left of pre-season, and got halfway through the season, and then I did it again. In a game. The same knee.

There was a ball in the air that came from my right side. I jumped off my left foot but with the wrong technique and didn't turn my body towards the ball. As I landed, I felt my knee shift, but still managed to kick the ball away. Play was still going on and so, I gently knelt down, and when I stood up did the 'can I stand on my leg and straighten it with control' test. I felt it shift again and was like, 'Oh no'. I yelled at my teammates to kick the ball out, and the physio came onto the field. I told him I thought I'd re-done it and he asked if I wanted to do the testing on the field or go in. I asked to be taken off so we made a sub and I went into the rooms.

The physio did the test and thought my knee felt really loose. I was pretty certain that I'd done it. He said, 'I know you have a World Cup next year. I think you should call your national team. We'll get an MRI in the morning'. He left me in the changeroom, and I called the national team doctor and coach straight away.

I was freaking out. The World Cup was only 11 months away. Soon after that initial call I went outside and sat on the bench. It didn't take long for the doc and coach to call back, telling me they'd booked everything and asking how quickly I could get things sorted to leave. The plan was for me to head straight to surgery, without going home to Canberra first. I would fly straight to Adelaide to see the same surgeon.

The MRI showed there was 60 per cent damage to my ACL. It was enough for everyone to decide it should be repaired. There was no other cartilage damage. I flew home a few days later, which gave me time to get organised and say goodbye to the team. More blood thinning injections were required again for the flight home. I also made sure I had a brace.

My knee didn't hurt much at all this time, but there was no stability. The first one really felt like something exploded in my knee, whereas this one just 'went'. There was a shift sensation, and then it felt really unstable. It did swell a bit, but not as much. I had three days in Adelaide before my surgery, trying to get the swelling down, even though there wasn't that much. All up it was around a week to ten days between me injuring my knee and having surgery.

This time around we used a patella graft. We also talked about using a cadaver graft, but because of the timeframe before the World Cup and my age (I was then 27) they felt a patella graft was the best option. It was strong and had a slightly different timeframe with the ability to introduce loading more quickly.

I literally woke up and started exercises straight after surgery. My physio said, 'Come to the side of the bed, we're doing magazine pulls!' We had no time to waste a single day. There was a definite timeframe we had to work with and a clear plan through the whole process. It was a bit more of a whirlwind experience compared to my first one. We were aiming to return to play in nine months.

I stayed in Adelaide again for the first week post op and had three or four sessions with the team doctor and physio. They outlined the plan—what I would be doing. Then I went back to Canberra. My rehab was to be done through the AIS, while still working with the same physio as the first time around. The rehab was run by the national team, and they spoke with my Canberra physio regularly. They worked well together in a really collaborative way. The email chain had around five people in it also including our strength and conditioning coach in Canberra, as well as my goalkeeping coach.

The rehab was more intense the second time for sure. The first eight weeks or so my mum had to drive me everywhere. We live around 25 minutes from the AIS, so she would drive me there and back for my two sessions each day. I'd be there from around nine until midday, then we'd go home, have lunch, and then return for a goalkeeper session where they had me catching a ball—while on my butt—for 30 minutes. That was my first three months of rehab before I could start running.

All of the national team preparation for the World Cup was being done in Australia. As soon as there was a camp, I was able to go even though I couldn't do anything. It was great to be a part of the team. Our national team physio was also able to do rehab with me on the camps and get a good look at my progress and what I needed to work on. Every three months I did dyno testing (a form of muscle strength testing) and had to hit a certain percentage. If I didn't hit it, then we'd stay there for an extra week of rehab.

At around the five-month mark, I would lunge and my ITB would flick over the outside of my knee. The pain was excruciating. My whole leg would go numb with pain and there was nothing I could do to stop it. It went on for a few weeks and we were all starting to get really concerned. It was at a critical time when we really needed to be amping things up, but I just couldn't because of the pain.

An ultrasound showed a boney growth under my ITB. Every time I bent my knee a certain way my ITB would flick over it. The theory was that when they were drilling for the patella graft, a bone fragment shifted and grew with the blood flow creating a bone spur in a not-so-great spot. I had another surgery in Canberra and they shaved the bone away. I only needed a week off, and after that the flicking stopped and I was back on track.

The World Cup was around 10 and a half months from my surgery. Return to play was planned for nine months. I managed to hit all of my timeframes and was ready right on time. My coach wanted me to play at least 10 games in the six weeks before the tournament for him to feel comfortable for me to play at the World Cup. I achieved that by playing every weekend in Canberra and midweek in camp, before we left for our pre-tournament in Canada, where I played another two games.

I felt comfortable with everything in terms of jumping, kicking, and diving. I had done controlled contact drills in my training, but I hadn't yet experienced contact in a game. There was definitely a bit of anxiety in each of my lead-up games. It was like I needed to get hit to know I was ok. It took until around the fourth game for me to feel confident with everything.

All was going well until two days before we played in the World Cup, when I strained my right quad. The decision was made for me to sit out the first game, but thankfully I was able to play the rest of the tournament, and my quad held up. We were also playing on turf, which was a bit of extra caution, as turf isn't the most well-liked surface. But I didn't have any knee issues throughout the tournament.

We came seventh at the World Cup. We were the first Australian team to make it through a knockout round. It was a pretty amazing tournament. And I couldn't believe I had made it there after 10 months of not playing at all.

My knee has held up well ever since. I've had some patella tendonitis in my left knee since the second surgery, but I manage it well. Kneeling still isn't comfortable, but jumping and landing are fine. I just have to take an extra 10 minutes or so to warm it up and load it before training. My knee prep work to this day has basically stayed the same, but I have a better understanding now of how it is all interlinked. I now realise, 'I need to do this' rather than thinking, 'The physios are telling me to do this'. Even if the other players don't do it, I still do. These days however, pretty much everyone I play with is on board with the ACL prep work and the education around it.

REFLECTIONS

The first time I did my ACL I didn't really know what was involved with the rehab. I didn't know how much it would hurt, or what it would mean for my career. I went a bit numb and blank to start with. The biggest thing

I was thinking was, 'There goes a year of my life down the drain'. I was in another country. I had no family or national team support near me. I wasn't even sure whether I was going home to get it repaired. It was all a bit daunting. The 10 days or so after the injury when I was still in Sweden consisted of a lot of organisational toing and froing, and that didn't really help my mental state. I wasn't sure what was coming next, let alone how I was going to cope with it all. It wasn't until more of a definite plan was organised that my sense of hopelessness started to lift.

My decision to return to Sweden for the end part of my rehab was due to a few different factors. It was the first time I had really been away from home and I was really enjoying my team in Sweden. I was only two months into my two-year contract, and I just didn't feel I wanted to leave. I was also at the age that I didn't really want to be at home. There was nothing really there for me, there were no teams to be a part of. I get a lot of my energy and sense of happiness from being around people. So even if all I could do by being in Sweden was to try to motivate and support the team, that felt like it meant more to me than just being at home doing rehab on my own. I knew physically I could do the rehab required. It was just that mentally I needed to be in a good place.

The second time was different. I literally had a day to cry about it, and a day to say goodbye to everyone, and then my focus shifted towards the World Cup. I was lucky to have one of the best players I've ever played with, Abby Wambach, reach out to me. Abby was the top US striker in my team. She literally grabbed me on the second night and said, 'Don't worry, you're fine. Cry about it now, have a drink, and then tomorrow you can worry about rehab'. She was very experienced and motivational and believed in herself so much. She just gave me so much positivity about it all.

After that I never had a doubt I couldn't succeed. Even when I was getting the bone spur fixed, the anaesthetist came out afterwards and said, 'You're one of the happiest people I've met!' I asked what she meant, and she said when they woke me up and wheeled me out to recovery, I had started clapping everyone and saying 'Thank you!'

The two rehabs had their similarities but also their differences. I didn't progress as quickly in Sweden as I did the second time around in Australia. It was obviously a smaller town so the quality of the gym, access to a dyno, and being measured with a tape measure rather than looking at true muscle density all contributed to me not really knowing where I was at physically in terms of my rehab. Mentally I felt good. But I guess the physical part was a little more relaxed.

Communication was also a lot more challenging in Sweden. It was the first time an Australian player had gone back overseas for their ACL rehab rather than complete it at home. I think it was relatively new for everyone as to how best deal with the communication involved and who had the right to dictate what needed to be done. Technically, since I'd done the injury at my club, and they were paying for it, Sweden had the right to run the rehab, especially once I returned. They were kind to let the national team take the lead. Despite the challenges, everyone worked well together, and we were lucky to have time on our side. I think as long as I was happy and healthy and doing the right things, then everyone was happy to be in that boat together.

Things were more streamlined the second time around at the AIS. I had everything they could throw at me leading up to the World Cup just to make sure that I was on the right path. It kept me busy, and motivated. I had access to the recovery centre, strength and conditioning, physio, a dietician, and a sports psych. There was always someone there to help me with any questions I might have had. There were also two other ACL-injured athletes, and a lot of AIS athletes around—it was inspiring to be in the gym and to see other athletes working really hard. I trusted everyone I was working with and I knew they were all communicating well. No one was over stepping what the physio wanted. No one was overstepping what the sports psych or strength and conditioning were doing. Everyone stayed in their lane.

Remaining an active part of the national team also helped immensely. I was able to go to camps, even when I didn't need to. I was still getting paid, even though I didn't need to be. Being around the team and involved in team meetings really helped me feel I was still a part of it all. Mentally that was so important to me. I think it was just as important as being given great physical rehab.

I wouldn't have changed anything with my second rehab. I had the right support around me, and was engaged and experienced enough to want to know exactly what the physical workload would entail, and how could I help to make it easier for myself and everyone concerned. If I could have my time again, for the first ACL I would have done a little more research into understanding what my rehab was going to look like, how it was going to work, and where the difficulties would lie. I was so concerned with my mental state, I think I just kind of zoned out with the physical stuff.

My biggest support through my ACL injuries would have to be my mum. My dad had passed away, so it was just the two of us. She was there for me at the very beginning of both rehabs, and dealt with my mood swings when I was at my lowest. I didn't think the first one was going to be so hard. Those first three months when I wasn't yet able to run was the first time that I hadn't been in a team environment since I was 16. Being at home without any outlet other than rehab was hard – for both of us!

A conservative approach for either of my ACLs was never discussed with me. I'm not sure what my thoughts on that would have been if it had been brought up. Interestingly I had a teammate recently who had a partial ACL tear and didn't undergo surgery. Her training wasn't the same afterwards, and she didn't feel as confident. She chose to get surgery later on.

I was on the pill both times when I injured my knee. I was using the pill to control my cycle around my sport schedule, and would come off it during the rehab periods. I am off it again now and haven't had any issues. I didn't track my periods then, but I do now and find that my energy levels fluctuate in line with my cycles. I wouldn't be surprised if my cycle contributed to my injuries, despite the fact I was on the pill, but the second one was definitely a wrong technique issue from me too.

I've certainly learned a lot through my knee injuries. The first one taught me how to take charge of myself and not leave it to everyone else to do. I learned how to take control. It was the first time I actually wondered if I was still going to have a career in football, and made me realise how fragile you could be with injury.

Second time around I discovered my body could do anything I put it through. I realised I needed to trust my rehab team as they were the experts, as well as trusting my body. When I first had to step down off a box to land, I felt I wasn't ready, but they said, 'Of course you are, you can do it!' I now know that no matter what I put my body through, it can adapt. I also understand my body a lot more now. If I'm a little sore I know I need to pull things back a little.

My ACL injuries have definitely made me more resilient, even though at times they've pushed me to borderline depression and despair. It is important not to overthink things, and resist the temptation to do more in pursuit of faster results. Rest is often the best thing for rehab or recovery.

ACL rehab means a long time is spent putting all of your effort and energies into one thing. I found one of the hardest things is when you're doing rehab, and you've done rehab for days, and it's only 10am. To have gotten through that month after month, it makes you realise that you did get through it, even if it was hard. That realisation in itself makes it easier to manage other stressful things in life.

Advice to my former self would to be more open-minded to the people who are coordinating your recovery. To listen to what they have to say. When I was younger, I was a bit stubborn and hard-headed as I hadn't had anything serious happen to me. Doing my ACL the first time bought me down a level, and taught me to appreciate the people who don't get enough gratitude and recognition for how hard they work behind the scenes for athletes.

Advice to others? As everyone says it's not the end of the world. If you can look at it in a positive light you will get through it. You're not going to be in that spot forever, and you will come back from it. You will recover. It might change the level you play at, or it might not, but you will get through rehab and return to play or whatever it is you are doing. Just try not to be frustrated with not seeing results straight away. As soon as you get frustrated you will lose sight of the actual goal, which is you being able to perform again.

NETBALL

KIM GREEN

Kim Green is an Australian netball player who ruptured her left ACL towards the end of her career. Her reconstruction—utilising a hamstring graft—and rehabilitation were conducted in Australia. After surgery she returned to play what she considers to be her best netball.

I started playing netball when I was eight and was picked up professionally at age 15. My career included 14 years of playing with the Sydney Swifts, before moving over to captain Giants netball in 2017 for my last three years when they became a new club within Netball NSW. I also played for the Diamonds—Australia's national netball team—for nine years before retiring from international netball at the World Cup in Sydney in 2015. My career highlights include winning Commonwealth Games gold and silver and two World Championship titles with the Diamonds, and four premierships with the Swifts. But we don't collect medals or trophies in our house, so whenever anyone asks to see a medal, I don't know where they are! I really just played netball for the love of it.

Growing up I played all sorts of different sports. Mum was an Olympic swimmer, and Dad was a footy player, so I've come from a sporting family. I was a happy-go-lucky kid who loved being active and playing anything, anywhere—it didn't matter what the sport was.

Never did I ever think I was going to be a netballer. I always thought I was going to be a running athlete. I was a national sprinter and hurdler in my early teens, putting my time and effort into trying to qualify for the World Junior Championships. Netball was just a fun hobby on the side.

With my speed and power, I started being selected for state netball teams. I then received a phone call randomly from the Swifts coach, asking me to train with the team to boost numbers on court for pre-season match play. Being just a young kid who loved playing, I didn't see it as a door to an opportunity; I just thought, 'Okay, I'm just going in to be a number, off I go'. I played a couple of quarters and was called back to do it again the following week. After that second session I received another phone call about signing a contract with the Swifts. I realised then what a great opportunity it was, but to be honest I had no idea who was even in the team other than Liz Ellis and Cath Cox, whom I'd seen on TV.

The tricky part was that I wasn't able to do athletics and netball. I had a really strong think about it with Mum and Dad, who essentially put it back on me saying, 'Do what you love'. When I really thought about it, netball was where I felt happy. Athletics put a lot of stress on me, being an individual sport. After that I made the decision pretty quickly and said, 'Yes, I'm going to take this opportunity'. My athletics coach was very upset with me, but ultimately understood. And the rest is history in terms of my netball career.

Netball is a tough sport on the body, especially on the lower half. I have had my share of injuries and niggles throughout my career. My first couple of ankle sprains occurred when I was younger playing basketball, and then

I badly sprained my right ankle at a netball Nationals. I have accessory naviculars (an extra bit of bone on the inner arch of my feet), and when I tore all the ankle ligaments it ended up protruding even more afterwards. Later in my career I had a stress fracture in the right accessory navicular, and a left lateral shin compartment issue. I also hyper-extended my right knee and partially tore my ACL a couple of years before I tore my left. The partial tear completely healed—it was just a little nick of the ACL which repaired itself.

My left ACL injury happened in 2017. I had just moved to the Giants from the NSW Swifts, a huge emotional rollercoaster. I knew many fans weren't going to be happy with the change, and I had always wanted to be a one club player. The time for change had presented itself and I embraced it. In a full circle moment, the same coach who picked me up when I was 15 came back to coach the Giants. To start and finish my career with the same coach was just too good an opportunity to refuse. I knew she would be able to bring out my best, as well as nurture me as I approached the back end of my career. I was made captain of the Giants, and we were creating a new club from the ground up; that was something I'd never been a part of. It was really special. I had new teammates and a renewed zest for life.

We were playing in Canberra in round five, and I was the fittest and strongest I'd ever been. I was feeling so good going into the game. We were coming up against one of the lower-ranked teams, which is often a harder game because you know it's going to be more physical with some rough bumps and bruises. Within the first 10 seconds of the game, the ball was down the other end but coming back our way. I dodged and drove for the ball, caught it, and then turned as my opponent made impact on me from behind. Straight away I felt something go inside my knee and there was a 'pop' feeling. It felt like my whole knee had rotated inside—it was like something had happened that shouldn't have happened. It was a disgusting feeling. There was instant pain, but 20 seconds later it was gone.

I had to be helped off the court and into the changeroom. I could feel my leg didn't have a whole lot of stability. The doctor confirmed on the spot that my ACL was gone. So many thoughts were going through my head, 'It's the backend of my career'; 'I'm just starting with a new club'; 'We were going so well and it was so exciting, and now this'.

Immediately I messaged my mum who was in the crowd. Straight away on my phone a twitter notification popped up that read: 'Green's gone down with a knee injury, there goes her career'. I thought, 'Jeez, already?! Thanks people!'

The decision for surgery was made really quickly. At half-time I was in another room because I didn't want the girls seeing me upset as they needed to finish the game. The doctor said, 'These are your options, these are the people, I'll get on the phone right now and try to book you in'. Then my coach came in and suggested we go with a particular surgeon who'd done a lot of knees of netballers, and the doctor agreed that he was a great option. I had no idea, so was just happy to go with their suggestions.

I saw the surgeon two days later. He confirmed it was my ACL and outlined my options. He said he normally used a hamstring graft for a netballer but asked if I had any thoughts on other graft types. I was happy for him to use whatever he thought was going to help me get back out there and perform to my best, so we went with the hamstring option. He had mentioned patella grafts but said that they could lead to irritation and interference with patella tracking for netballers. That was really the only other option he discussed. He didn't use synthetic grafts.

It was 10 days before I went in for surgery. I had some bone bruising that needed to settle down which caused the delay. In the meantime, I had activation and strengthening exercises to work on. I was lucky to have a clean ACL tear and no cartilage damage.

The nurse had me up straight away after surgery trying to teach me to walk up a little step. My hamstring was not having a bar of it! I was thinking to myself, 'Why is she making me try to get up a step when I've just had surgery? Do we have to do this right now?!' But I understand now she was just trying to make sure I was safe to go home from hospital!

Another player was picked up to play in my position for the Giants. She actually came to live with me in Sydney. She was not only the perfect person to fill my position at the Giants, but also to nurture me through that time as well. She'd done two ACLs, one on either side, so was such a valuable person to have around. I was really fortunate, because she looked after me so well, and made sure I didn't do anything that I shouldn't.

I was tracking really well at the beginning of my rehab. Rehab was every day, three times a day, and I was achieving good quads activation and building up my muscles nicely. I had two different physios working with me—an experienced AFL physio, and a new team physio who had some previous experience with teams from the Northern Territory. Having two physios had its benefits, but was also quite conflicting at times. One physio was telling me I needed to start heel-to-butt hamstring exercises while lying on the floor, while the other insisted I shouldn't do any open chain exercises, referring to the surgeon's post-surgical orders. I was so confused—I didn't know what I was supposed to be doing.

At around three months when I was completing the testing to determine if I was allowed to run, another communication breakdown occurred. One of the tests was an elevated single leg bridge, but I hadn't progressed to that yet. I had only done elevated double leg bridges or single leg bridges from the ground. I mentioned this, but was told, 'This is the test'.

So, I did it… and then 'pop'. My hamstring tore. I knew straight away. I didn't have pain. It was a strange feeling, but I knew something wasn't right. But the physio said, 'You'll be right, you'll be able to run'. I did a bit of super-light running on the Altar G with 20 per cent of my body weight. But as soon as I got off, I knew it wasn't right.

I'd lost faith in the system, not knowing who was right and who was wrong, or what I was supposed to be doing. Not having one physio stamp their authority on my recovery and rehab was hard. I felt I needed one person to be driving it. In the end I called the Diamonds' physio, someone I trusted totally and with whom I had worked with previously. She didn't want to step on any toes but helped clarify what I should be doing. She suggested a scan, but I declined as I felt I knew what I'd done, and that it should be enough just to rehab it.

I kept chipping away and building my hamstring back up. But it was so slow. It would cramp trying to get my heel to my butt while I was standing and brush my teeth or with simple bridging exercises—and that was four months down the track. I just wasn't building any strength.

My strength and conditioning coach worked really well with the Diamonds' physio. They had some great programs up and running for me. I was due to head over to Los Angeles for 12 days for a business trip, and I was lucky to be able to take my S&C coach with me to continue my rehab. It allowed her to see how much my hamstring struggled with everyday things like going up steps and getting in and out of the bus we drove, not just in the gym. She knew I was doing all of my exercises correctly, plus more, and could see something wasn't right. She said: 'As soon as we get back, you're getting a scan'.

When I finally had the scan, it showed I'd torn my graft site and it had never reattached. I had torn through my scar tissue which is why it probably didn't hurt when I did it. Being one hamstring down explained why my hamstring strength just wasn't improving the way it should have been!

We then had a shift in personnel within our medical team. We worked with the Giants AFL physios in the interim, but they were so busy with their own athletes it wasn't ideal. I ended up finding a local physio and finishing my rehab there. That meant I didn't have to drive out to Olympic Park every day in Sydney traffic which was becoming extremely draining. It was off season, and everyone else was travelling around the world doing great things, and here I was every day for five hours rehabbing. It was a very testing time mentally. But I'm glad it was happening to me and not to a younger player.

Once we figured out the hamstring issues, my S&C coach created a program that allowed me to get some sort of activation within the hamstring. I started to show a lot of progress. But there was still a

30 per cent difference in the strength between my right and left hamstring, when it was approaching time for me to get back on court. Because it was such a long way off the five per cent difference we were aiming for, I went back to see my surgeon. When I asked the risk of me doing it again, he replied abruptly, 'High. You're working off one less hamstring'. He then asked my reason for wanting to come back when I was at the back end of my career. Was it for fame? 'No'. Money? 'I don't get paid enough to do it for money!' Then why? 'I just love playing'. To which he replied: 'Just go out and play then!'

It was a relief to hear it didn't matter what that final percentage difference was, as long as I could get it to be close to my best. We just had to change the end goal line and bring it a bit closer to my hamstrings' new reality. There ended up being a 30 per cent differential when I was playing. The closest I got was 18 per cent. I just found other ways to hide the deficit, as athletes do.

As soon as I'd had the last conversation with the surgeon, I felt like it was time to get on with it. 'Let's just get it done.' I was like a bull at a gate, but my S&C coach was running my return-to-sport program and was making sure I didn't overdo it. Because we were in off-season, we weren't pushed for time, so I was able to have some game-play practice before the season started. I was able to get back to playing within 12 months.

I didn't have any mental blocks when it came to returning to the court. Bracing was never an option in netball, and I felt 100 per cent confident in my knee when I returned to playing. I had no fear of doing my knee again, because I had done so much work, building every other muscle in my leg knowing my hamstring wasn't right. I just knew I was going to be fine. And if I wasn't, then I was never going to be. I was perhaps a bit more mindful initially of how I landed after body contact—I remember going 'Uh!' for a moment with the first big knock. But then I jumped back up and was fine and didn't think about it again.

Even before I did my knee, I used to do a lot of activation work to get prepped and warmed up before games. But after my ACL I became very particular about my pre- and post-game prehab/rehab and was far more diligent about it. It was all targeted around my hamstring and I had a very systematic way of preparing before games and trainings—I didn't like anyone messing with that routine. I also took pickle juice throughout the games because I continued to cramp in my hamstring, and that seemed to do the trick for me.

Despite the hamstring deficit, I came back and played my best netball. To this day I don't have any pain in my knee. I have full range of motion, it's just my hamstring that remains a bit weak.

REFLECTIONS

My ACL journey showed me that my body could do so much more than I thought it could. It's funny that Twitter told me straight away that my career was over, but never did I think that. I remember on the way home from Canberra wondering to myself, 'I know I'll be okay, but is this the right thing I should be doing?' I guess I was looking for a sign of some sort. We were driving up the highway and two double rainbows formed. I'd never seen a double rainbow in my life, let alone driven through one for five minutes straight! It was amazing. And I just thought right then and there that was a sign I was where I was supposed to be, and that it wasn't time to give up just yet.

Soon after I'd done my ACL, I had a couple of athletes reach out to give me advice. That was really lovely. The one thing they all said was don't compare yourself to others who have had knee injuries. And I thought, 'No, I won't do that'. But lo and behold, six weeks after the operation there I was hash-tagging 'ACL recovery' to see how I was tracking compared with others around the world! I think it's a natural thing to want to compare, but once I tore my hamstring, I realised that everyone's story is so different.

Mentally I was pretty solid throughout the whole process, although the changes in personnel and hamstring issues definitely tested me. But in testing times character is shown, and that leads to growth, and I definitely think there was growth for me.

I learned a lot about myself and my own leadership. I'd always thought I was a really strong leader, especially to young ones who had hurt themselves, or anyone who had a long-term injury. But I came to realise that I probably *wasn't* a great leader. I learned that what athletes with an ACL or a long-term injury need is constant support throughout their rehab year. They can't just have a whole lot of love at the beginning, and then little drip feeds here and there. They need people who are constantly there and consistent with their support. I think my leadership was strengthened from my whole experience.

Aside from the obvious setbacks, I think my ACL injury was the best thing that happened to me. I'd been playing for 15 years straight at that stage without a break and the injury allowed me to have some much-needed downtime. It also gave my body an opportunity to rest and recover and get itself ready to go again. I also realised that my body wasn't as flawed as everyone (including me) thought it was. Before the injury I had been tarnished with, 'Kim's got a lot of niggles, niggles everywhere', which no doubt contributed to the Twitter universe jumping to the conclusion my career was done for when I went down with the injury. Advice to my former self would be don't go on Twitter! The whole process showed me my body was actually in really good nick, it just needed a break. I think that break gave me a couple more years in my career at the top level.

The timeout also helped reaffirm for me that netball isn't everything. I had learned that a long time ago, but you do forget. It gave me a little glimpse of what a retired life without netball could look like, and I didn't mind it to be honest. It was refreshing. It gave me the time to put energy into driving my netball business and allowed me to have a great transition out of netball.

I'm not a sports psych kind of gal, although I was offered that service.

I tried really hard not to get emotionally attached to the issue after an injury, and to see it for what it is. I chose not to speak formally to anyone, feeling they may have pulled me into the injury a little bit more, and I didn't need that. But saying that, I do feel it is important to keep tabs on injured athletes. The contrast from when you're playing and everyone is in your corner and it's all about you, to when you're potentially no longer that 'athlete', is really interesting. It's like you become invisible, the attention stops, they don't even check in. That is something I always try to do now with anyone who's done their ACL: 'Just checking in, just saying hey, how are you going?' Regardless of whether they are an athlete or not, I think it's so important to keep touching base.

In hindsight, perhaps I should have listened to my gut a bit more in the initial stages. But when you're allocated a support team, you don't want to do the wrong thing by them. I'm not one to blame anyone for anything, but I was so unsure as to whom I should listen to and what I should be doing. I really could have benefited from experienced leadership internally within my rehab team, rather than having so many fingers in the pie. My S&C coach was my saviour. She knew I had an older body; she was the constant person that always had my back. I was fortunate to have her in my corner, and a coach who also knew my body pretty well.

The whole rehab process wasn't at all what I expected. Everything that had been prepped for me never happened. I was told it was going to be so painful after surgery, but I was off the drugs within a day. No pain. I was warned I would be so stressed when I got back out on the court, but I was never stressed. And that's why I just don't give advice, because if I told everyone that it wasn't going to be stressful and they weren't going to be in any pain, it wouldn't be correct for everyone. We're all different.

'Don't compare' would be my advice to others. Don't look at the hash tags. You don't need to. But no doubt you will, as everyone does… So, I guess allow yourself a peek, but just don't get caught up in it.

I don't believe there was a link between my injury and my menstrual cycle. My injury was due to a collision, and I was on the pill. But we do track our periods in netball and prepare more thoroughly at different times during our cycle.

If I tore my ACL again now, even though I am retired, I would go through the surgery again without a doubt. Everything on the other side of my injury was amazing. I played better netball. My body was better for it. It just enhanced my life. It really gave me a reboot.

RUGBY UNION

MITCH SHORT

Mitch Short is an Australian rugby union player whose ACL story is unusual. After sustaining a full ACL rupture to his left knee, he successfully returned to play just two weeks later. He then pulled back to complete a three-month block of rehabilitation and has since continued to play at a professional level. He has had no further issues to his knee.

I am an Australian rugby union player who plays in the halfback position. After initially getting my Super Rugby start with the Western Force in 2017, I returned to Sydney in 2018 to play with the NSW Waratahs, and Randwick in club rugby. In 2021 I signed with Paris's *Racing 92* in the French National Rugby League Top 14, and am looking forward to the opportunity to continue to develop my game at one of the biggest clubs in Europe. Being 26, I am hopeful my playing career has plenty more years to come.

Growing up I played rugby league, so was used to body contact and an oval-shaped ball. The school I went to didn't have a league program, so at around age 10 I found myself playing union. The more I played, the more I started to enjoy it. I also played some cricket during the summertime, but footy was always my passion—I was really obsessed with it. In year 12 (2013) I played with the Australian Schoolboys U18 team. From that experience I realised that playing professionally could be a realistic opportunity if I put my head down and continued that route after leaving school. And so that's what I did.

I started university part-time and focussed on training and trying to get a crack at playing for NSW. It paid off. I made it into the under 20s NSW side, and then after a stint in WA with the Force, I am happy to have ended up playing in NSW.

I managed to get through school sport without hurting myself. My first and only major injury before injuring my knee was when I was around 20 years old, playing first grade for Randwick—I fractured my right fibula. It wasn't displaced, so I was in a boot before starting rehab at six weeks. I missed between 10 and 12 weeks from that injury.

I did my ACL in my debut game for the Waratahs in 2018. It was round two and we were playing the Durban Sharks in South Africa. I was coming off the bench with around 15 minutes to go. Within the first few minutes of me getting on there was a lineout. I went through and got into the backfield and was sprinting at top speed. When I came to their full-back, I tried to step off my left foot. As I stepped, the full-back tackled me. I didn't feel a snap or pop or anything, and I got up from the tackle fine, but then, as I stood there for a moment my leg had this numb feeling. It went dead on me.

There was a break in play not long after, and I remember standing in the scrum wondering if there was an issue in my knee. My leg was a bit shaky, and I didn't feel great. But with all of the adrenalin, and the fact I'd only been on for a few minutes, I didn't spend too long thinking about it and managed to play on for the last 10 minutes. In that time, I felt fully capable and was still taking off, running at top speed, and surviving tackles. It was only when I was jogging during slow parts of play that it felt like something wasn't right. But I wasn't too concerned and went on as usual. I even managed to score at the end with my first try which was pretty special. All the more so when I found out later that my ACL was actually no good!

After the game, I had to do some top up conditioning. This is a bit of fitness work to make up for the fact I hadn't played the early part of the game. I'd cooled down for a few minutes before starting, and when I went to take off again, I could just feel it a bit in my knee. I flagged it to our trainer and was sent into the shed to see our team doctor. I explained to her where the feeling was, and what had happened on the field. I didn't know what the ACL test was at the time, and so when she did the test and said it felt a bit loose, I didn't think much of it.

I was so stoked at having played my first game and wanted to make sure I was ready for the next week. I iced my knee heavily with the Game Ready ice machine, but that night I was in quite a bit of pain.

The next day we flew to Argentina for the second game in our two-week tour, and my knee actually felt quite good. The pain had gone. We landed in Buenos Aires on the Monday, and the medical team checked it again and thought it might be a good idea to get it scanned while we were there. The scan happened the next day, and it revealed I had torn my ACL.

Despite the results, I could still pivot off my left leg and I felt confident on it. I was trying to prove to our doctor that I was good and able to stay, but she said it was too much of a risk. She couldn't guarantee I would be physically able to play big minutes if the other half-back went down. I was sent home on the Wednesday, and that was it.

I'd gone from the highest of highs playing my first game and finally being in the team I wanted to be in, to flying home the next day. I wasn't happy.

I was in an interesting head space on the plane. I knew surgery was probably a reality, but I was keen to see if there was another way of treating it if possible. My contract was up at the end of the year so I was keen to avoid having surgery straight away if I could. I wanted to be fit and able to prove I could play games to try to secure another contract the following year. But I also knew that this was a major injury, and although I was keen to keep playing, I was concerned about causing future damage to my knee down the track. I didn't want it to shorten my career.

Once home my knee kept feeling better day by day. There wasn't really any major swelling, and after that first night, the pain had gone. Our team doctor returned from Argentina the following week, and considering how well my knee was presenting so soon after injury, was very open to the conservative option. She described other successful cases, and the team physios and other medical staff all did a lot of research on the topic. I was keen to avoid surgery, because I knew if I went down that path I was definitely out for the whole year.

Later that week we saw a specialist for a second opinion. He looked at the scan, and then at my knee, and said, 'You've definitely done it'. He didn't feel there was any point re-scanning as he could see enough already. There was some bone bruising, but no other cartilage damage. I explained my situation, and that I was keen to give conservative treatment a go; deep down I felt I could make it work. He agreed that treating it non-surgically could be an option, but was a little more hesitant than our team doctor as he hadn't seen it done successfully before at the professional sport level.

It seemed no one was telling me I absolutely had to have the surgery. I made up my mind to go with the conservative option. My plan was to get off my knee for a while and not train, and then build it back up slowly through a full rehab process.

The following week there was another injury to the other half-back player at the Waratahs. That meant they were effectively down to no one—we were all injured! With the way I had been describing how good my knee was feeling, it was put to me a few days out from the game if I wanted to give it a go and try to play. There was no pressure to say yes, as they'd get someone in if I didn't feel okay about it. It obviously wasn't only up to me—our team doctor was a key part in the decision, but I jumped at the opportunity. To me, it seemed like my best chance to put my name forward to secure a contract for the following year.

Up until that point I had been doing physio exercises but wasn't doing any formal running or gym program. I was staying on top of my VMO and quads function and doing lots of single-leg balance work and things like that. Once they suggested I could play, we strapped up my knee and started putting me through fitness tests over the next few days involving changes of direction, ball skills, and contact. If at any point I didn't feel it was safe or smart for my knee, our doctor was ready to make the call that I was unfit for play. I had to tick off everything before they would let me play. They were giving me until kick-off to prove myself, and other half-backs were on standby in case I didn't make it.

I was pretty confident in my knee and passed all the testing. It didn't once feel like it would give way on me. I trained with the team the day before the game and was able to complete that without any issues. I progressed through all my kicking and was cleared to play. It was unreal.

After doing my ACL in Durban, I was playing again two weeks later! I was strapped up heavily, mostly at the back of the knee as I didn't like having tape all the way around. Running and stepping felt okay, but I was a bit tentative with contact early on. I think it was more of a mental thing. I knew I'd done my ACL and was aware of what usually happens—which isn't playing rugby two weeks after the injury, but I settled into things pretty quickly and stopped thinking about my knee about 10 minutes into the game.

The plan was to play for 50 minutes and we stuck to it. I believed I could have stayed on longer, but we were ahead in the game at that point, and with everyone just a little unsure about my knee, it was deemed best for me to come off.

I pulled up well the next day and stayed on the icing regime. I came into the club on the Monday feeling pretty good and started to get all of the VMO and hamstring stuff firing up as I thought that would give me the best chance of staying stable.

My knee was doing fine, but I was back playing off the bench after another half-back returned from injury and took the starting spot. There I stayed for those two games, playing only short stints. Then the Wallabies half-back returned as well, and once he slotted back in, it meant I was out of the team.

We then discussed going down the conservative management path properly and giving my knee the complete rest it required. We also had the knee rescanned to see if there had been any more damage. It showed there was still a bit of bone bruising, and our doctor explained we wouldn't know if it was from the initial injury or from me running. Surgery was mentioned again, but I was still keen to try the conservative path. If it didn't work out after three months, I was prepared to get it fixed surgically.

After that we pegged everything back and I completed a full rehab process over the next 10 to 12 weeks. I stopped running for the first few weeks, but stayed the course on the strength side, and slowly built back into running and change of direction. We kept adding bits and pieces along the way until I returned fully to play. It felt pretty good. I was confident throughout the process that everything would be fine, but I definitely benefited from having that time off and strengthening everything around my knee.

I returned to training with the Waratahs, but I wasn't being picked to play. I played for my club team at Randwick for the remainder of the year (eight games). I was signed again for the Waratahs for 2019, and although I had a few stints on the bench, didn't really get on the field again that year so I continued playing at Randwick. I was re-signed again in 2020 and played five of the six games until COVID hit. I started for two of them and played off the bench for the other three.

I strapped my knee early on, but by the back end of 2019 I stopped the strapping. It's continued to feel really good since then and I haven't had any instability episodes. I'm well and truly back to normal. I do everything in the gym and on the field, and I haven't missed a session.

No one talks about my knee anymore. It's been good to move on and get back to normal. I don't worry about it at all. To be honest, I haven't thought about it for years!

REFLECTIONS

I learned a lot from my injury, particularly around listening to differing opinions and being open to alternatives. I'm lucky my knee was a bit different. I almost feel bad telling my story as it is so much shorter and seemingly easier than most others who have gone through an ACL reconstruction.

ACL injury management seems to be often presented as a one option scenario—that being surgery. And that too was my assumption after my scan in Argentina. At the time the only option I was familiar with was surgery, and then six to nine months of rehab before returning to play.

If our team doctor wasn't as open to non-surgical management, I am certain I would have been just like everyone else. 'Yep, I've done my ACL, off to surgery straight away'. I probably wouldn't have even asked too many questions. But she talked with me about the options in great detail and outlined stories of others who had returned to play without an ACL. I had heard of guys playing without their ACL, but they'd all ended up getting it done at a later date, or their knee had completely gone on them. If it wasn't for our doctor, I definitely would have had the surgery.

I can't deny there was a big cloud of doubt hanging over me. Being only 21, and at the very start of my career, I was a bit unsure if what I was doing was really in my best interests. I was worried about not only surviving in the short term, but also of doing damage that could shorten my career down the track. And there was also the risk of it failing after 10 or 12 weeks. I can't say I didn't wonder at times if I was just wasting time trying to manage it conservatively. I was also aware of the potential negatives to having surgery—that you can re-rupture, or do the other side. I just didn't want to jump straight into it.

I had only a few moments of knee instability—if I was lazy in the way I was walking or if I stepped on an uneven surface. It felt like it would hyperextend a little and cause mild jarring at the back of my knee, but it never fully gave way or made me fall over. They were only minor episodes that happened a handful of times up until around three months after the injury. To prevent it I quickly realised I had to be really good with my VMO control in the gym. I found that my leg weight work really helped.

My medical and rehab team was really good. They recognised what I was doing throughout the whole process, and could see that I was capable. I didn't really have any major setbacks along the way. If I ever felt pain, I would stop and be smart with my training. The only thing I changed was to not squat too deeply when carrying heavy weights for around the first year after injury. If I jumped the gun with weights and got carried away, my knee would swell a bit, so I became really strict about how I did my weights. Now it's not an issue, and I no longer worry about my range.

I still stay on top of my VMO activation and quads strengthening work. Before I hurt my knee, I didn't work at it as hard as I do now, and definitely didn't do my prep work before training and games anything like I do now. I always feel good if I'm putting load through my leg and keeping my quads in synch.

I can't really fault my rehab process. My biggest issue was I was just frustrated and so badly wanted to get back to playing. It felt weird having played a game and been training for a few weeks, to then pulling right back and having to stop. That was my only complaint really, that I had to completely stop. But I believe it was smart the way I built back up and I became more aware of the role things like hamstring strength play in being functional. I couldn't do Nordic hamstring curls straight away, but once the bruising settled and as soon as I could do the movement, I started to feel quite good. There is only a slight strength deficit now, but not more than 10 per cent—I make sure I do my hamstring work to stay on top of it. I'm glad I wasn't rushed into surgery to have my hamstrings potentially interfered with for a graft.

When I look back, I don't think I did anything silly that predisposed me to doing my ACL. My training was well-rounded, and I was happy with the way my body was functioning before the injury. Initially I thought the injury occurred due to the contact of the tackle but looking back I think it must have been the pivot, as the tackle just didn't look like the motion where you do your knee. As to what made that pivot different to others that I'd done thousands of times before, who knows?! Injuries are part of sport, and I think that for whatever reason, it just happened. I just really didn't want it at that time in my career!

Others in the team who had done their ACLs were most interested in what I was doing. They would watch me and just shake their heads. Maybe jealous? I'm not sure. I was just lucky with whatever it was—the strength around my knee, or the way that I run, or whatever—that I could cope.

I don't have the magic answer to which knees can 'cope' without surgery and which ones can't. It's so individual. But I think there are more knees like mine that aren't given the time to prove themselves.

My advice to others who have suffered an ACL injury is to be open to other people's views. Listen to your specialists and seek more than one opinion so you can be sure when you make your mind up as to what's best for you and know your body and be in tune with it. I believe you can tell if something is really right or not if you listen. Trust your body and be smart with what feels right and what doesn't. Don't just be dependent on someone looking at a scan and telling you what you should be doing. Having your own opinion about your body is important. If you don't think your ACL injury is too bad for you personally, I feel you should explore conservative management as an option.

Whichever way you go, whether that be surgical or not, be disciplined with your rehab and your training, and get yourself in the best possible physical shape. You have to give yourself every chance to get fit again.

FREESTYLE SKIING

ANNA SEGAL

Anna Segal is a professional freestyle skier who has undergone five knee surgeries in her career—four ACL reconstructions (one to her left knee, and three to her right) utilising three different graft types (hamstring, cadaver, and quadriceps tendon), and one arthroscopic 'clean out' (on her left knee). She has experienced surgical management and rehabilitation in Australia and Canada, as both a self-funded aspiring athlete and fully supported elite athlete. She has also competed with and without a functioning ACL.

I am a professional skier who competed in freestyle skiing for 14 years. Born and raised in Melbourne, my skiing career began at Mount Buller, where I worked my way onto the Australian moguls development team when in my teens. I then moved into slopestyle—skiing down a course and doing tricks over features such as rails and jumps—and spent most of my twenties competing on the slopestyle world circuit. During that time,

I won X Games gold, silver, and bronze, made numerous Dew Tour podium placings, and, in 2011, was awarded Australian snow sports person of the year after winning World Championship gold.

I retired from competition after placing fourth at the Sochi Winter Olympics. I then transitioned into the world of backcountry skiing. Now based in Whistler, Canada, I am still lucky enough to make a living through my skiing via film parts and photographic shoots.

Skiing has definitely given me my share of injuries over the years. I've had a right ankle reconstruction, broken wrists, a stress fracture in my back, four concussions, a spiral fracture of my middle finger, and a broken thumb which now has a plate in it, as well as lots of other bruises, bumps and sprains along the way!

All up, I've had four ACL surgeries. The first was in 2005 when I was on the Australian moguls development team. I had just finished year 12 and skiing had been on the back burner while I completed my studies. After working diligently at my school work and going hard in the gym, my light at the end of the tunnel was that I was taking the next year off to ski. My plan was to try to get onto the World Cup team, and to qualify for the 2006 Winter Olympics.

I travelled to Canada for my first training camp, and two weeks in, while landing a 360 degree jump into the moguls, I blew my left knee. I don't remember if I felt a pop, but it was a clean ACL rupture with no other damage. It was the first big injury I'd had and I was devastated. I remember my coach tearing up. He was a big guy and seeing this made me feel as though my skiing was over. My world came crashing down and I was full of self-pity, 'Why me?', 'I'd worked so hard', 'I'd pushed through year 12', 'I'd gone to the gym'. It was really hard for me.

I flew home, had surgery, and started uni. Hobbling around campus on crutches wasn't the best start to uni life. Everyone else was out partying, meeting friends, and having fun, while I was rehabbing, and just trying to keep the swelling down in my knee.

My first knee reconstruction used a hamstring tendon graft. I had quite a conservative surgeon who was recommended by my mum (also a medical professional), and he really held me back from doing anything full-on for a long time. I wasn't allowed to run until six months had passed, and I wasn't allowed back on snow for 11 months. Everything was slowly progressed. I think because of that conservative approach, my ACL healed really well.

As a younger athlete I didn't have much of an inbuilt support network. My physiotherapy was paid for out of my own pocket. Initially I had a strength and conditioning coach from NSW's Institute of Sport (NSWIS) writing my gym programs but living in Victoria I didn't have face-to-face access. When I decided halfway through my rehab to quit moguls and focus on park skiing (slopestyle), it meant I was no longer part of NSWIS, so no longer had that support. I was out on my own.

I started working in a ski shop at around five months after the surgery. The job had me on my feet for around eight hours a day. On top of the rehab, the work really inflamed my knee.

No physical testing was conducted to determine when I was ready to return to snow. From my physio and my surgeon, it was more of: 'It's been 11 months and you've been working hard. You should be good'.

At the end of the year (2005) I went back to North America. I was given guidelines by my physio on how to return to skiing progressively, but he didn't have a background in winter sports, so I had to figure most of it myself. I did three weeks of groomers, then started to build up slowly. Really, I was guessing as to what I should be doing. I was wearing a brace, but it wasn't a good one and I ditched it about a month in. After six months of skiing my knee felt good. Nothing hurt. I didn't notice it anymore. I felt good. I felt strong.

My next ACL injury—on the other knee—occurred at the start of 2007. I'd had a good stint when I was knee-injury free, and I don't believe the two injuries were related. I was now skiing slopestyle, and had just won my first big international competition. I'd beaten all of my idols, was being interviewed by the ski magazines I'd grown up reading and had lots of sponsorship contracts and amazing travel opportunities coming to me. I was on top of the world.

I was in the terrain park working on my tricks. I had a new confidence in myself that I just hadn't had before: 'I'm good, I'm going places!' I was trying to land one particular trick, but I was tired. I just kept going and going and going. I didn't have the sort of coach who would hold me back, or anyone telling me to stop. It had been a long day and I probably should have called it. I landed heavily from the jump in a big rut in the snow, and my body kept twisting once I'd landed. I felt more than just a pop—it felt like an explosion. It was the most painful knee injury I've had. It was excruciating.

My surgeon told me it was like a 'bomb had gone off' inside my knee. I had torn the patella tendon off the bone, and had ruptured my medial collateral ligament (MCL) and ACL. In surgery they again used a hamstring graft, but also stapled my patella back to the bone, and stitched up my MCL. There was a lot of swelling and heat in my knee after that surgery.

My physio told my Mum I probably wouldn't ski again, and if I did, I definitely wouldn't be competing. But he never told that to me. He kept my rehab really positive, but at the same time, he never pumped any false hope into me. He knew I wanted to return to skiing, and he never shot down that idea for me. He just said we needed to be really conservative, and told me what I would have to do to get there.

Despite the second ACL being a far worse injury that the first, I knew the process ahead. At the three-month mark when I was allowed to get back in the gym, I hired a trainer as I believed that was what I needed. I worked really, really hard at the gym, and churned out a good 10 months of rehab—again.

The rehab was similar to the first, except swelling was more of a problem for me this time, and often held me back in the gym. My trainer wasn't with me for each session—initially it was once a week, and then only once a month. I remember that being a bit of an issue as I pushed through swelling and pain without having anyone to tell me to rest. There was also more pain due to the extent of the injury, and so progression was a little slower. It took me longer to be able to squat, and do any single leg work.

Mentally, I dealt with it better. I knew if I trusted the process and ticked off all of my rehab, then I would be okay in the end and get to where I needed to be. It was still pretty tough, but I was able to work through that more easily the second time around.

Uni held me back from returning to snow too early, as I had to finish my exams. It was around nine months after surgery when I was able to return. This time I wore a custom-made brace when skiing. I then started to wear two braces, one on each knee as I felt I just couldn't let this happen again. I wore them until the end of my competitive career.

My knees behaved themselves for the next few years and I was skiing well. I was regularly on the podium and loving life. Then in 2013, I had an accident competing in a World Cup; I chipped off a piece of cartilage in my left knee. I thought it was just a meniscal tear, but woke up after having an arthroscope to be told I'd punched a huge hole in my articular cartilage. The surgeon didn't do a microfracture during surgery, because we hadn't discussed it beforehand and I had the Olympics coming up. He just cleaned it up as best he could and decided to try and let it heal.

It was tough as I was constantly in pain, but there was nothing I could really do about it. My knee had constant swelling, and no-one could tell me how long it would take for the pain to go—or if it would ever go. I was given a timeline that would have me back on snow in three months. But when I did return, I couldn't even turn my skis properly because I was in so much pain. It still hurts me today if my muscles are tired and I'm out skiing—I still feel pain where that cartilage is missing.

That injury really messed with my confidence, as I would always anticipate pain on landings. Always coming out of a trick and knowing you were going to be in pain is not a good way to be in your head. I was really struggling. My left leg was weakened by the surgery, and there was the chronic pain I was continually working through. I think that probably contributed to my next ACL injury on my right leg.

I don't exactly know when I did my third ACL—there were a few incidences when it most likely partially tore. I was competing in a World Cup again, and wasn't feeling very confident. I rushed myself back onto snow because the 2014 Olympics were coming up, but I hadn't been competing or jumping very well. It was in a snowstorm, and I was trying to get my tricks back as quickly as possible so I could practise my run before the Olympics. I landed a trick on the tail of my ski which hyperextended my leg, and I felt a bit of a tweak. My physio checked it out, and I took some pre-planned time off over Christmas. The back of my knee didn't feel great, but I thought it was just my hamstring.

When I returned to training after the break, I did a trampolining session to help regain my air awareness and practice my tricks. Landing from a jump I felt a click and instant heat in my right knee. It wasn't excruciating pain, but it didn't feel right. I stopped jumping, and went to see my physio. She did all of the standard knee tests, and I caught a look on her face that wasn't good. She was concerned and sent me to get an MRI. I immediately thought, 'Oh no, something has happened here'. I went off and got the MRI and was told I had five per cent of my ACL hanging on—in other words, it was hanging on by a thread. This was three weeks before I was to leave for the Sochi Olympics. After all of the issues I'd had rehabbing the left knee in the leadup, now I'd torn my right ACL. It was pretty devastating.

Luckily, I had a really amazing team behind me. I had a fantastic coach, physio, and sports psych who were all working together to do whatever they could to get me to the Olympics. With three weeks to go I didn't have time to get surgery. We did whatever it took to get my knee in the best state possible to get back on snow and then we'd see how it went. That was all we could do. I felt if I could try, and it worked out, then great. If not, we would have done everything we could.

My days were filled with conditioning and recovery, as well as a lot of mental preparation. My sports psych had me getting up in the morning, putting on my ski gear and lying in my bed visualising for up to an hour.

Then I would use the Pilates reformer at the physio, then lunch, then to the gym for gentle muscle-activating exercises with my physio and coach. I had eyes on me at all times. Anything that was too much they would make me stop. Everything was progressed very gradually so as to not aggravate my knee. I would then do pool recovery to help with the swelling and mobility, an evening physio session, and then ice, elevating, and resting.

I also put a lot of effort into my diet with as much anti-inflammatory food as I could. I ingested a lot of green tea, turmeric, ginger—anything I had heard was anti-inflammatory! I was doing everything I could do to get my knee into the best shape considering what had happened to it.

Just before we left for Russia, I was allowed to return to snow to ski some groomer runs. It was designed to be easy—I was to ski five runs just to see how my knee reacted to being in ski boots and skiing. A few days later I was allowed to go into the terrain park and hit three jump lines to see how my knee felt on landings when it was all strapped up. It didn't feel great, but I passed the tests and was allowed to head off to the Olympics—albeit with a big question mark over my head. That question mark felt even bigger after we inspected the Olympic slopestyle course and discovered it was absolutely massive. The jumps, rails and features were the biggest I'd seen in competition. Bigger than X Games. Bigger than any World Cup course. It was just huge.

I passed the additional physical testing for the Australian Team to let me compete once I arrived in the village. At that stage I was just happy to be there. I wore my two knee braces, and before skiing each day my physio would heavily strap my knee so I couldn't fully straighten it. The tape made it a little hard to get my grabs and perform everything I needed to do, but my knee felt really safe. Training was a fine balance between slowly trying one feature and trick at a time, while keeping my total runs to a minimum so as to not aggravate my knee. Once off snow each day, it was a structured schedule of recovery, visualisation, physio, and ice baths.

I completed four training sessions on the course before competition which helped to increase my confidence. But I only had around 50 per cent confidence in my knee. I tried to put it out of my mind. I figured if I lost, my knee was already blown. But if I won, then awesome—I would have competed at the Olympics and put down a run. I felt I didn't have too much to lose.

I qualified into the final, which I didn't expect. I placed fourth overall, which, with a blown knee, I also didn't expect. I think it goes to show the power of mind over matter and the importance of having a really good support team around you that you can trust.

After the Games I flew back to Australia and went straight in to see my surgeon. Having already used both hamstrings previously, I was out of luck there for graft choice. The patella tendon on my right side was not in good shape having already been torn, and the only other two options were using the patella from my left leg, or a cadaver graft. We chose the cadaver graft, thinking the patella graft would potentially cause me too much trouble in the future. I had to choose between two types of cadaver graft—one that had been treated with radiation, which had a better chance of being accepted by my body, or one that had been cryogenically frozen and had a better chance of bonding well. I chose the cryogenically frozen graft.

The third rehab was so much quicker than my previous two. I was able to get back into the gym and start strengthening work a lot sooner because I didn't have to wait for the graft site muscles to heal. There was a lot less swelling, and a lot less pain. Overall, the rehab went surprisingly smoothly compared to the others.

My first day back on snow was ski touring at six and a half months. It was a little early, but I had two knee braces on, and kept things really mellow. Doing my first turns out in the Australian back country was definitely not your average return to snow protocol! It was right for my new direction in skiing—I had stopped competing and was aiming to spend most of my time ski touring (using my skis to walk up the mountain) and filming jumps in the back country.

Over the next few years my knees were great. I was skiing a lot of powder snow, and I was jumping less. In 2017 I decided not to ski with the knee braces anymore. I found them quite uncomfortable for ski touring, and believed my knees were strong enough to not rely on them anymore.

Everything was going great—until I decided to jump again. I was working at a free-skiing and snowboarding summer camp on Blackcomb Glacier at Whistler. I got a bit excited and decided to start hitting the big jump (60 foot) and get back a few of my old tricks. I came up short on the landing and felt no pop or click, but my knee just hurt. I thought, 'This isn't good'. As soon as I could get down the mountain, I went and saw the physio. She did the usual knee tests and told me she thought I'd torn my ACL again. MRI confirmed she was right—the cadaver graft had torn.

It took me a month to get in to see a surgeon. It felt like an eternity after being used to seeing my surgeon in Australia pretty much immediately. And that was only after a fellow Canadian professional skier called her surgeon on my behalf. Thanks to my friend, I got an appointment a few days later, and was on the operating table soon after that. It's a little bit about who you know sometimes which is really unfair I think, but for me it was lucky.

For ACL number four, we had a really long and positive discussion about the best graft option. I wanted to continue my skiing career for the next few years, and the surgeon didn't think another cadaver graft was the best idea. He thought it would probably blow again because I was clearly in the habit of really pushing my knee. His idea was to take my quadriceps tendon from my left leg to use as my right ACL graft. He thought taking my right quad tendon would further weaken my already damaged quad/patella. He used a 10 millimetre-diameter chunk to really beef up the graft, as well as help fill my ACL tunnel—which, at that point, was quite large due my previous surgeries.

The pain during my recovery from that quads-tendon graft was really intense. I found the graft site on the left leg was a lot more painful for the first three months than my ACL injured leg. I would be up at night with it throbbing. I couldn't squat for a long time. It didn't swell, but it just killed me with the pain. A friend suggested I try THC and CBD oil (cannabidiol oil or medicinal cannabis) and it was the only thing that helped. I hadn't had that kind of pain with the hamstring grafts.

My rehab was different this time because I didn't have a strong or favoured leg. Both of my legs were pretty weak, and both were in pain. I couldn't do a lot of the quads building work initially because of the tendon pain, and so they both really atrophied. But once I got over that, at around four months, things went ahead really quickly. Because I didn't have a leg to favour, I felt more stable and my squatting came back more evenly than in the past. I also think my balance was better. I remember, with my hamstring grafts, my balance was really off.

I was back on snow in six and a half months—pretty quickly really. I kept things really mellow and followed a return-to-snow protocol that defined how many runs I should do a day, how many days on, how many days off. I really stuck to that. I had to do a photo shoot with one of my sponsors 10 days after I was back on snow, but I told them my skis weren't leaving the ground. I stuck to my guns and all I had to do was a few turns for the camera. I was doing a lot of ski touring, which allowed me to be out in the snow, but I didn't have to do as many runs. I was also doing a lot of cross-country skiing, and a lot of time in the gym. There was no specific timeframe that I needed to be back for this time, so I was more patient than previously. Again, I kept things mellow—as hard as that was! I think that was better for me in the long run. I didn't start jumping until around 10 months after the surgery.

I decided not to wear a brace this time. I knew if I started to wear one, I would just have to wean myself off it again. Braces were great for me when I was competing in slopestyle, with the high impact I had to put my knee through every day, but I didn't believe I needed them for ski touring—which is essentially walking up hill much of the time. My aim was just to build up all of the little muscles in my knee to ensure it was as balanced as possible, and to get back on skis without a brace—and to stay on skis for many years to come! So far, the plan has worked!

REFLECTIONS

It's interesting to reflect on all of my ACL injuries and where my head space was during each one, and all of the things I have learned. I have definitely taken away a lot of life lessons through it all. That first knee injury was definitely the hardest. It wasn't the worst injury—it was actually the most typical of all of my reconstructions—but mentally I had no idea what I was in for. I didn't realise how long the rehab would take, and I'd never had my physical ability taken away from me before. That was really tough for me.

I knew I would be able to ski again, but there were a lot of unknowns. I had no one else to share stories with or tips to help me mentally. No one else I knew had done it so it was hard to know what to expect and not knowing is always quite scary. People were sympathetic, but I didn't get much empathy. My mum didn't know what I was going through, and I didn't haven't any ski friends around me when I was rehabbing to tell me their stories. I had no one telling me the little tricks and tips like trying acupuncture or taking an ice bath after training. I was figuring it out all by myself and relying on my determination and willpower to get me through. Mentally it was quite draining.

In hindsight (having learned from three more surgeries!) I should have picked part-time work where I was off my feet. I think that set me back and made my knee swell for longer than it would have otherwise. When I see others who have had ACL surgeries and are waitressing or working on their feet all day, I always think, 'Uh uh, you need to spend your on-feet time in the gym, and the remaining time you should be focussing on recovery'.

Before my first ACL I thought I was invincible. I was young and didn't know what a proper injury was. I didn't realise I would have to overcome mental challenges. Getting back on snow and having what could happen in the back of my mind definitely messed with my confidence a bit. After learning how to tackle that, I used it to my advantage with the subsequent injuries.

The second time round, I knew more friends from slopestyle skiing who had injured their knees. I realised I wasn't the only one it had happened to—it was actually quite common in my circle. Also, having gone through it before, I knew what to expect. I'd learnt a few tricks along the way to help me and I knew the rehab timeline well. I knew the benchmarks I needed to aim towards, and I could pace myself better mentally to get through it.

When I had the cartilage removed in my left knee and was trying to prepare for the Olympics, I moved to Sydney just for rehab. I was definitely over-training—I was training six days a week, at least two sessions a day, three sometimes including Pilates, and was surfing on my days off. I was so obsessed with the idea that 'more is better'. I believed the more and the harder I trained, the quicker I would be back on snow, and the better I would be able to ski, but it went completely the opposite way.

There was also conflict between my strength and conditioning coach and my physio. My S&C coach's approach was 'harder is better', and working through pain was a good thing, because if I had to do that in competition then I'd be well prepared mentally. My physio's approach was that too much could actually take me backwards—she felt my knee swelling up was my body's way of trying to tell me something. And if I wasn't listening to it, I could be doing more damage than good. I was torn as to whom I should listen to, which was really hard.

I learned some important lessons from that scenario. If you have a team around you, they need to communicate well together; and going harder isn't always better. If you're training so hard you can't do the next training session, then you're doing too much. Slower progression is also better than just pounding your body and thinking you're superhuman, because your body reacts adversely to that.

After my fourth ACL surgery, I applied those lessons from my pre-Olympic journey and got some amazing results. I was lucky enough to have the Canadian snowboard team's newly appointed S&C coach agree to work with me, and I trained with him at the Canadian Sports Institute satellite gym in Whistler. His approach was different from what I had experienced in the past. He urged me to do less and come in the next day fresh, rather than overdo things and be too sore to do anything. It was a less goal-orientated approach than I'd had previously. If I was ever sore, he would always tell me to stop. I'm one of those people who likes to tick off all of the exercises on my list to make myself feel good, but if I was sore doing one of the exercises, he would tell me I was done for the day and would pretty much send me home. I'd never had that before. That slow approach to the rehab helped me a lot.

Once I was able to get back in the gym, I progressed really quickly. I just wasn't sore everyday like I had been in the past. Because my S&C coach was stopping my workouts when they needed to be stopped, the knee didn't really swell much as it had previously. In the end, it got me back to strength and onto snow really quickly. Importantly, I wasn't stressed when I was rehabbing the fourth time and I was sleeping really well. During the other rehabs, I was either at uni studying and doing exams, or I had a lot of pressure on me to get to the Olympics. I had really high anxiety levels which I think affected my recovery badly. With my fourth ACL I wasn't under a whole lot of stress professionally, and I was able to sleep well. I was working mostly from home, and if I needed to go to bed early I could. Each day I would wake up feeling refreshed.

My injuries taught me a lot about risk evaluation. This is important when doing something dangerous is part of your career—weighing up when it's worth it, and when it's not. I also learned about training smarter, not necessarily just training harder, especially as I became an older athlete. I was more efficient with my training, rather than just training more, and knowing when to stop. But mostly I learned that if I set my mind to something, even the toughest situation, I could get through it. I think it taught me a lot of grit.

Conservative management wasn't discussed as an option with any of my ACL injuries. It didn't feel great skiing without my ACL in the Olympics; I didn't feel I could perform to the high level I needed. When I did sharp turns on the slopestyle course at the Olympics, I could feel a big shift in my knee when I applied force through my skis. It was definitely my preference to reconstruct the missing ACLs. I felt it was important for me to have the best ligamentous support to protect my knees from further cartilage damage.

When my professional skiing career comes to a close, I still want to be able to ski, surf, climb, and trail run. These are the things that make me happy in life, so I want to make sure I am still able to do all of those things into my later years. For me, the nine to 10 months of rehab is worth doing for the ability to do all of the things I love. But saying that, I do have friends who are managing to ski well and choosing not to reconstruct their knees after recurrent ACL ruptures.

It is hard to say for me whether my menstrual cycle could have been linked to my ACL injuries. My cycle can be very irregular. I have also been on the pill at certain times too. But I am aware that there is research out there showing increased risk of ACL tears at certain times in the menstrual cycle. But for me I have never tracked my cycle or given it that much thought. Maybe I should!

If I could offer advice to my former self, it would be to watch my energy levels and take more days off to rest. Don't push through fatigue, especially when trying to learn new tricks, as that's when you're most likely to injure yourself. And there's always tomorrow to achieve your goals if your body or mind isn't where it needs to be on a particular day.

If I could go back in time, over-training was the biggest thing I would change for my first three injuries. I also wish I had discovered THC/CBD oil earlier. I used it on my quad tendon site and it really helped with the night pain.

Advice to others would be to do your research to find a good physio. Get recommendations for a sports physio who works with athletes and ACL injuries, and has experience returning athletes back to their sport. Physio is a broad profession, and you want to find someone who specialises in what *you* are trying to achieve and invest in a good trainer to get you back to where you need to be. Physio gets you so far, but then you've got another chapter of strength and conditioning you need to do.

AUSTRALIAN FOOTBALL

DANIEL MENZEL

Daniel Menzel is a former Australian Football League (AFL) player who sustained four ACL ruptures—the first to his right knee, and then three to his left—during his professional career. Reconstructive surgery was undertaken in Australia for each injury, initially utilising two hamstring grafts, then a LARS graft, and lastly a patella graft. His rehabilitations were also conducted in Australia, with a short training period with a USA-based conditioning specialist during his final rehab.

I played AFL for 10 seasons after being drafted to Geelong in 2009. I played as a forward with the Cats for nine years, and then with the Sydney Swans for my last year, in 2019. I played 80 AFL games, but missed many more than that due to injury. I unfortunately underwent four ACL reconstructions. I try not to look too much at the negatives and more at the positives. At 28, I returned back home to Adelaide and continue to play and coach in the South Australian National Football League (SANFL).

I haven't hung my boots up yet.

I played a range of sports when I was younger, but AFL footy was always my number one. Having five brothers, my love of the game initially came from playing footy in the backyard and just developed from there. AFL was the sport I always hoped to be successful in.

Before I was drafted to Geelong, I had osteitis pubis. I had issues with my groin and core as a lot of young footballers do. Other than that, I didn't have any major injuries before I entered the AFL.

My first ACL was my right knee in September 2011. I was 19 and in my second season with Geelong. I had played three senior games in my first season, and had a breakout season in my second, playing 18 games. We went into finals in second place on the ladder, with every chance of winning the premiership. The week before we'd played the top team, Collingwood, in the last round of the year, and beaten them by 16 goals. I kicked five of those goals and received the three Brownlow votes that day. I was playing well, full of confidence, and thinking we had every chance of playing in a premiership in three weeks' time.

In the qualifying final against Hawthorn, I started the game really well again kicking two goals. In the second quarter the ball was going out of bounds, and I ran after it, with my opponent in close. We were hip and shouldering each other as the ball went out. My right leg caught between his legs, and we twisted. My knee didn't really have anywhere else to go and my ACL ruptured. That was the start of a long, long journey ahead for me.

There was a very obvious pop. I went down holding the back of my knee. There was agonising pain for maybe 30 seconds, but then the pain went completely. They stopped the game and I was stretchered off the ground and taken down into the rooms. The doc wasn't 100 per cent confident initially I'd fully ruptured my ACL, so I asked if I could just run up and down the changerooms to see how it felt. I think they knew things weren't great in my knee, but they let me do it. I struggled to decelerate with my stride throughs and realised I might be in a bit of trouble. Within those few minutes my knee blew up a fair bit. They sat me back down, had another feel, and said they were pretty sure I'd done my ACL. And that's when it hit me. All of the emotion. I knew what an ACL injury was, and I knew the timeframe that went with it. My finals campaign was over.

I went in for surgery a week later. The thinking behind getting it done so soon was so I could return to play as quickly as possible the next year. There was no other damage, it was just a straight ACL. The two graft types discussed were patella and hamstring, as the surgeon had experience with both. There was a chance the patella grafts could cause patella tendonitis, so we chose to go with the hamstring.

After the surgery I was at home icing, doing my exercises, and managing the pain. I definitely wasn't pushing things. But after a couple of days I woke with intense pain during the night. It was worse than the pain of doing the actual ACL, and I couldn't escape it. My knee had swollen so much I had to see the surgeon again to get it drained. He drained two full syringes of fluid. The relief was incredible. It was better than any pain medication I'd been given. Although the setback was small, the pain was immense and led me to be not such a fan of short timeframes between an ACL injury and time of surgery.

My rehab was pretty standard for an AFL player after that point. It was your typical three months to start running, six months to start training, and around nine months to start playing. We followed weekly plans and didn't have too many hiccups along the way. It was probably my most straightforward rehab.

I felt confident in the people around me. My physios were all very experienced and I had access to a great conditioning coach. We ticked off all of the jump landings, twisting, tackling, and uncontrolled contact in the air. They were the main things I felt I needed to tick off mentally to be prepared. After completing them in training, I'd then complete an extra week of it, so I'd be able to build even more confidence before playing.

It was soon after nine months that I returned to play. I was pretty good to go. Nerves were always going to be there, but I didn't go out feeling unsure about anything or thinking I just needed to get through the first game. I had no taping, as I didn't believe it would do much for me. I went out trusting I would be okay and be fine to play. I was confident we had ticked everything off.

My first game back was with Geelong reserves in the Victorian Football League (VFL) in July of 2012. Someone kicked me the ball and I was running on a lead at a decent speed. I bent down across my body to pick up the ball and it felt like someone pushed me from behind and my left knee gave way. It was a very similar feeling to my right, with a definite 'pop' again, and similar pain. But it didn't make sense. It was the other knee! I went down to the ground and was stretchered off. Straight away my thinking was I'd definitely done something again.

My usual rehab team weren't at the game. There are different doctors and physios at the VFL and AFL. They were happy to wait for my usual doctors to confirm what was going on rather than jump straight to it, even though everyone was thinking it could be my ACL. When I did see my usual team later that afternoon, they thought it was pretty similar to my first presentation. The replay showed I didn't have any contact from behind like I thought, so that was bizarre. But they were all pretty sure I'd done my ACL.

Once I realised that I'd done it again, I broke down. My initial thought wasn't about playing, or getting back, or career longevity, it was purely, 'I'm going to miss out again on another premiership'. The team had gone on to win that Grand Final in 2011, meaning I missed becoming a premiership player by two weeks. My driving force every single day during the past months of rehab had been to win the premiership the next year. And that goal was now empty.

I saw the same surgeon, and we chose a hamstring graft. I hadn't had any issues with that graft on my right side. This time we took an extra week or so and I made sure the swelling was right down before heading into surgery after what had happened the first time.

The plan with my rehab was to again take nine months. This being my second ACL, and me being a professional athlete (a driven one at that),

I felt I could be right in eight months this time. I was pushing the limits and knew where I could get ahead by a week or two here and there if I did everything right. We had everything on track and going well. I was around a week ahead at each stage.

It all came crumbling down at the six-month mark in December 2012. I was doing a controlled tackling drill with a coach—I tackled and they twisted, and I felt a small 'pop' in my left knee. It was only subtle. I felt I'd just twisted it awkwardly. We had a new physio at the club taking my rehab that day, and although I felt okay to keep going, he called it there and made me go inside just to make sure. We went in, and he felt my knee. He didn't think it felt unstable, but it didn't feel awesome either. As he hadn't rehabbed my knee so didn't know what it normally felt like, he said, 'I can't rule out you haven't done your ACL'. Straight away I got emotional. He suggested we go in for scans.

The scan was somewhat inconclusive. It showed a definite ACL tear, but they weren't sure of the extent of the damage. I went back to the same surgeon, and he initially thought my knee felt strong enough and that I might be okay. He said he'd look at the scans closely over the next hour and get back to me later in the day. Just as I was about to leave for Geelong, our team doctor rang saying, 'Good news! From what I can see you haven't torn your ACL'. I was ecstatic, so ended up spending a bit more time in Melbourne thinking I didn't have to go straight home now. I left my phone in the car, and when I returned to drive home there were a couple of missed calls from the doc. I called him back and he said, 'I'm so sorry mate, the surgeon has had a look at the scans and thinks you have torn your ACL'. I bawled my eyes out the whole drive home to Geelong.

I was battling mentally at this stage. Geelong is great in the fact that it's a one-club town, and everyone gets around you. But that also becomes its own weakness for players, because the exposure and spotlight on you is huge. Everyone knew about my knee—it was well documented and talked about. I didn't think I could handle everyone asking me about it again, and I felt if we told the playing group it would definitely leak out to the public and media. We decided to keep it within our network until we knew exactly what we were dealing with and had a plan to move forward.

That strategy worked well until a few days before the surgery. The players knew I'd had the incident on the track but didn't think anything of it because we hadn't said anything. When one of the senior players came up to me in the physio room and said, 'Mate, good news! You're all good to go!' I was as flat and frustrated as anything, and remember swearing and saying, 'You've got no idea! I've torn my ACL'. It was like someone had died with his reaction, he just kept saying, 'I'm so sorry'. And that's when I knew we had to tell the club.

When deciding about the surgery, my physio and I had a big discussion. He felt there were two options, as we wouldn't know the extent of the damage until the surgeon went into the knee. If my ACL was more than 50 per cent intact, maybe it could be left, or a LARS graft could be used. If it was more than half torn, then it at least needed a LARS or a traditional graft. I made my decision off the back of mental factors more than physical. I'd just done back-to-back rehabs and didn't feel I could do a full third one. Physically yes, but mentally no. In my mind we had to do a LARS due to its shorter rehab time. I couldn't do a traditional graft again and be out for another 12 months.

We ran over the options with the surgeon. If he'd had his way, he would have done a patella graft, and the club probably would have agreed. But I was sold on the fact that if a LARS graft failed, we would only lose three months. It was a bit of naïve thinking from me. The surgeon hadn't done any other AFL players with LARS, just a volleyballer. But he was happy to try as at least one AFL player then had reported success in coming back after three months, so there was proof it could be done. My decision was made. I went in for surgery just before Christmas of 2012. I had torn 75 per cent of my graft.

The rehab didn't go well initially. I started getting severe headaches, and the team doc sent me straight to the hospital. It turned out I had meningitis. Probably because I had also decided to take the opportunity of the time out from training to get my wisdom teeth out, the week before my knee surgery. My body had taken a fair whack. That set me back a few weeks with my rehab, so the three-month timeframe was already blown out to four which wasn't ideal.

When I jumped into the rehab, I was shocked at how quickly I was able to do everything with the LARS. I didn't have pain, and I could move and progress so much more easily than with my other rehabs. The only thing that we implemented more of this time was gymnastics-type exercises and jump landings on safe surfaces. I had always done this in the past, but this time it became more than 50 per cent of my training.

I played my first game at 18 weeks, enough time for a LARS graft. It was the first time I had made it through a game in a couple of years, but the following week in my second game back, I did my fourth ACL in 19 months.

It was the second quarter again. All of my ACLs have happened during the second quarter! I was running directly at my opponent. He changed direction to run around me, feinting to go to my left, then right. I reacted and stuck my left leg out, then went to twist back to my right, and my left knee just gave way. It wasn't really painful, it just felt like something had given way and my leg felt weak all of a sudden. On the replay it looked so innocuous, but just showed that the LARS graft didn't hold up to a stressful movement.

The trainers came running on and called for a stretcher. My exact words were, 'I'm not being f***ing stretchered off the ground again!' The ball went over my head as play was still live, but I just didn't have a care in the world for it. I was so angry. I walked off the ground and, as I entered our rooms, I punched the door in frustration. I found out a week later I'd fractured three of my fingers, but obviously that was the least of my concerns.

The VFL physio and doctor were with me again. I knew I'd redone it, and they did too. By this stage I'd learned to expect the worst. There was no sugar-coating it. The AFL team were playing interstate and got back to our rooms maybe an hour or so later. When they all walked in, I remember looking at their shocked faces and I was thinking, 'What have I done, putting everyone though this again'. I couldn't even bring myself to call my mum. I didn't want to tell anyone because I just felt like I'd let everyone down again.

By this stage I was the most known player in the AFL for doing my ACL. When I went for the scan the radiologist called to suggest using the back door as there were a lot of media people outside. I was pretty over it at that stage, but figured I had to speak to them at some stage. I said I'd talk to them after the scan, which confirmed the ACL had gone. Their questions were predictable, 'Is your career over?' 'What are your plans from here?' I replied: 'I don't think you can say over, but I'll talk to the club to see what we can do about it.'

We gave it a few days for everything to settle and to think over things. My mum and brother flew over to have a meeting the following week with the coach, physio, and head of football. I was very lucky that Geelong was going to stick by me. Knowing that took a huge load off my mind. The plan was to spend two weeks searching the world for the best surgeon and researching lots of different cases to find out the best way back from this. I don't think the medical team could have planned any more for an ACL than with this one. There was so much that went into it.

After looking at all of the specialists around the world, the recommendation was another Melbourne-based surgeon. We met with him and I couldn't have been more impressed with the person he was, or his examples and his cases on different players. I was very much engaged in the whole process at this point and he answered all of my questions and was really down to earth. I walked out feeling that going with him was absolutely the right move for me.

We booked in another meeting for a few weeks to go through the plan. I didn't know the extent of it at this stage, but he said, 'It's going to have to be two surgeries. And it's not going to be a nine-month rehab. It's going to be 12-15 months at least'. The scaffolding holding the LARS in place had to be taken out, and the resultant holes in my knee filled with allograft (donor) bone fragment. Once that had healed—after three months—another ACL graft would be put in. I obviously didn't have any hamstring grafts left, and as quads weren't a big thing at the time, he suggested using a patella graft as he'd had success with them and felt they were as good and as strong, if not stronger, than hamstring grafts. Their main downside was potential patella tendonitis issues, which I did unfortunately experience later on.

I realised I wasn't going to play for the rest of that year. Or the year after. That hit me a bit. Mentally it was tough. But I was happy with the plan he gave me and confident it could work.

As I couldn't train for three months after the first surgery, I took a well-needed mental break and headed to Europe for five weeks. With no ACL graft in there at that time, I couldn't tear it or do any damage. Although I didn't feel all that strong or stable in my knee, it coped well with the holiday, and I was refreshed and ready to go when I came back. Mentally it made a massive difference to me as it broke up the rehab.

My rehab went really well until the running stage at three months. I kept getting patella tendonitis in my knee which caused me a lot of trouble. I would be so sore that everything I did took a couple of weeks longer to progress through than it should have. I couldn't kneel on my knee at all, and anytime I knocked it on a table I would be in excruciating pain. As I couldn't shake it, I had a CT scan that showed a bone spur at the graft site on my patella. The surgeon shaved it back in another surgery at around the nine-month mark, but I still had patella tendon pain in my knee for a good few years after that.

I was fortunate enough to train with a conditioning specialist in the US for 10 days. I had worked with him previously during my first rehab and was hoping he might be able to help with my tendonitis. He couldn't fix it, but he did help it. Because of his training techniques, and how diligent he was at getting everything activated and working together, it took a lot of stress off my knee. By the end of the sessions my knee would feel pretty good, but once it would get cold again the pain would come back.

My return game in the VFL was in July of 2015, effectively 30 months after my fourth reconstruction. I played six games in the reserves, and then had a rest week, before finally making my comeback in the seniors, against Collingwood—1450 days since my last AFL game. Coincidentally, playing against Collingwood was my last full senior game before I'd first done my knee.

I played well kicking four goals, but it was a weird night. We needed to win to make finals with only two games remaining of the season. For me every year my goal had been to win a premiership, so as much as I wanted to come back, I walked off the ground that night after we lost by 48 points pretty shattered. I didn't know how to feel. I was a bit emotional and remember saying to my physio, 'I'd give all of my four goals if we could have just won the game and just play finals'. He just looked at me and said, 'I know you don't realise it just now, but you've got to take a moment to understand what you've just achieved'. Then all of my friends and family came walking in and it was as if we'd won the Grand Final the way they were reacting. And that's when the magnitude of it all hit me. I was extremely happy. And proud. And thankful.

I continued to play with Geelong for the next three seasons. I played most games with some pretty good footy in there. But I continued to battle with ongoing knee pain, which in turn led to groin soreness. I had around 10 cortisone injections into my groin over those years to get me through playing. And I was playing at 80 per cent and could barely do half of my weights program. The realisation came that I was a compromised athlete, that I'd never be able to just train and play and be a normal person or player; it was a constant battle.

At the end of 2018 I decided I needed a change from Geelong. I moved up to Sydney to play with the Swans. They gave me new scans for my groin and put me in for a new groin surgery where my pubic joint was stabilised with mesh, as well as an adductor release on my left side. I felt amazing after the surgery. I felt normal again, which I hadn't felt for seven years. I was really optimistic about Sydney and was aiming to play in round two or three, but then I tore the adductor on the left side the week before. I didn't play until round 11, against Geelong! At the end of the season, after I had played seven senior games, the club wasn't quite as close to winning a flag as they had hoped and said to me they were looking to go in a younger direction. And that's how I found myself out of the AFL.

I moved back to Adelaide to play and coach at the SANFL level. I played with my brother Troy at Centrals, and then in 2021 we both moved to Woodville-West Torrens. That gave me the opportunity to compete for a premiership, finally. In October 2021, 10 years after my journey with resilience and adversity started, I played my first senior Grand Final. We won by 67 points! I finally felt as though my body was letting me perform the way I wanted it to. I kicked four goals, and my brother three. To come full circle and win a premiership, not at AFL level, but at SANFL level which is still an incredible standard, meant every bit as much to me as I hoped it would.

My body has never felt better. I finally feel what I would describe as normal. I don't feel like a joint-compromised athlete anymore. And that's one of the real positives out of it all for me. Although playing with Sydney didn't work out long-term, they fixed my groin and that's something I definitely needed. And as my knee surgeon said, 'For someone who's done four ACLs you're as lucky as can be to have not had any cartilage damage'. At the moment and into the future I don't think I should have too many more issues.

REFLECTIONS

Although filled with hardships, my ACL journey was an incredible experience. It was a real learning curve for me, both physically and mentally. Looking back, I think it took me until my third and fourth rehab to really nail it. Although I would have loved to have been on top of it all a bit earlier, I guess that's one of the bonuses of doing four!

So many people said to me along the way, 'Why would you keep going?' I had a lot of motivational factors that drove me, and one of my favourite quotes of all time sums it up, 'Pain is temporary. It may last a moment, a week, or in my case a few years. But if I quit it will last forever.' That stayed with me during every game I watched from the grandstands.

In my mind the toughest thing about an ACL injury is the length of time involved. It's hard to get your head around. Straight away your season is gone, and you've got to look to next year, and that's extremely challenging for anyone who plays competitive sport. Also knowing the magnitude of the rehab to come, and how much work you have to do, that's what hits you. Even more so when you've done that work already and you've still re-ruptured. It's just so hard to comprehend. I almost think your first ACL is the easiest one, as you're a little bit naïve and don't really know what you're in for.

Many professional athletes put on a persona during long stints of rehab to avoid showing weakness. I didn't want to bring down others around me or put extra stress on them by saying I was struggling or needing help. I remember thinking, 'I'll be able to overcome this. I'm strong. I'm going to struggle, but I've just got to deal with it'. That approach just builds up pressure over time. One of my teammates actually said to me during my fourth rehab, 'If you don't tell us what you're going through mate, how are we meant to help you?' That really hit home, and spurred me to stand up in front of the whole player group and explain where I was at mentally, and in what situations I struggled or when I found things more enjoyable. Opening up released the pressure I'd placed on myself, broke down barriers, and changed the conversation. Guys no longer walked away from me or acted awkwardly not knowing what to ask. That made a massive difference and mentally had me in a much better position.

I did see two sports psychologists during my first and second rehab. They were good, but I didn't click with them and found their techniques didn't do much for me. But by the time I was in my fourth rehab, my persistent patella tendonitis eventually led me to see another sports psych. This time

I really clicked with him. After I'd explained my situation, he asked, 'So when do you think about your knee?' My reply was, 'It's never not on my mind. I go to the shops and have 10 people ask me about it here in Geelong. There are premiership posters in every café. In the club I have my teammates ask me about it every day. It's in the papers. And I'm rehabbing, so I train on my own away from my teammates which is a reminder I'm not the same as them'. Then he asked about other activities outside of footy. I replied, 'I don't play golf anymore because I'm afraid it will hurt. I don't go to the beach because I'm worried a wave will knock my knee and I'll hurt myself. When I bend down in the shower I think about my knee and making sure I don't slip.' And he was like, 'There's no escape is there'. With that he explained that although I did have tendonitis in my knee, the anxiety I'd built up around it was so incredibly high, I simply couldn't get past it. He suggested we try a few different practices and see what would happen. He wanted me to watch my surgery video while my knee was sore so I would feel the pain while watching. I was to watch Geelong's Grand Final win, and look at the premiership posters.

It was extremely difficult at first. He also wanted me to play golf and go to the beach. Everything I was worried about he wanted me to do. If it was making my knee too sore, I was to stop and just think, 'It didn't work today, but I'll try it again tomorrow'. Within two weeks, the pain in my knee had gone down by at least 50 per cent, and I was able to nearly fully train. I was shocked at how much of an impact that could have.

That experience also really taught me to turn to things you enjoy doing when things aren't going well. Particularly when you're going through a long-term set back, whether that be injury- or mental health-related. In my first couple of rehabs, if things weren't going well, I'd go home and write off the day. But one of my physios said to me, 'Don't let a bad session turn into a bad day'. Which was a great point. By my fourth rehab, I had lots of other things in place. I coached my own under 14s team, did a lot of commentary work, and completed further study. So whether I'd had a good or bad day at the club, I could put that aside for the rest of the day and forget about my knee. It meant my life didn't just revolve around my knee.

I also put a lot of unrealistic pressures on myself along the way. I remember writing down and saying to myself that my fourth ACL was going to be a perfect surgery and rehab, and my rehab template would be viewed as the one to do by anyone who had done their ACL. That was all well and good in theory, but I was setting myself up for failure because every time I had a setback, and I had many, it would hit me like a tonne of bricks because I would think, 'How are people going to look at my rehab now and say it's the perfect rehab?'

Because no one had come back from four ACLs before in AFL at that stage, my journey was well documented. My story was picked up by Fox Sport and made into a documentary. At that time no AFL player or club had done such a documentary, so I was extremely nervous about how it would be portrayed. But once it was released, I received hundreds of messages from people who had done their knees, or had mental health issues saying, 'I can relate', or 'Thanks for sharing, it's helped me through my journey'. As a result, that was the start of my website and business Mental Toughness Mental Fortitude (www.MTMF.com.au) around resilience and overcoming setbacks and injuries.

I never thought the documentary was going to have the impact it did. Although I'm grateful it was received so well, it probably put even more pressure on me. I'd proved everyone wrong who said, 'You won't come back from four'. But then that changed to, 'You're not going to be the player you once were'. So that became my next challenge and goal. I wanted to prove to everyone that no matter what happens, you can still be a better player and better person than you were pre-injury. And I battled with that for the next three to four years.

My rehab journey had a lot of setbacks, but it forced us to work out ways around them and correct my deficiencies. I am more powerful and balanced even now than I was pre-injury, and there are things I can do in the gym that my teammates can't because I've done them forever. And those are the sorts of things that on the back end of my career make me a much better player. Although at the time I thought my rehab wasn't going as well as I would have liked, now that I look back on it, it shaped me in a really good way. I still do activation exercises before each session to get everything working together, and I feel like my hamstrings, glutes and quads get more bulletproof with each repetition. Those habits will stay with me forever now.

I don't think there's anything we could have changed in my rehab program that would have stopped my left ACL from going, aside from time. Maybe if I had given myself an extra two to three months on top of the first rehab, then my story might have been different. I try to pass that on to others now. What's another few weeks or months in the scheme of things? Doing one ACL is bad, but it's not going to be a problem for the rest of your life. But it will if you keep re-rupturing. So, give yourself the extra time you need.

Time was also responsible for my decision to do the LARS graft. If I could go back, I wouldn't choose LARS. But saying that, my brother successfully returned from a LARS at 16-years-old and went on to play for Carlton and Adelaide. He has to be one of the longest surviving LARS success stories, now at 25, because in the AFL, the majority of them have ruptured.

Hindsight is a beautiful thing, but I don't really look back and go, 'What if...?' I don't think it's healthy. Without the setbacks I wouldn't have discovered a lot of the things I learned along the way. When you go through a lot of challenges and stress, and your body gets put through a lot of pain, you realise how much you can actually push yourself. And that's something that I now always fall back on, I know that I can withstand a bit more than most.

Trying to play without my ACL was never seen as an option for me. AFL is such a demanding game requiring so much pivoting and turning, I don't think it would work. Even if in years to come we realise that it is a viable option in the AFL, I wouldn't sit there wishing I'd tried without. I'm just not wired to think that way.

The advice I would give to my former self would be to learn as much as possible from those around you. Listen to everything they have to say. If they're putting time in for you, they're only doing it to help you. Also, just because people haven't experienced exactly what you're going through, don't judge them because of that. People can't necessarily understand it, and you can't expect them to.

You need to lean on those people around you. Even if they can't actually help you, it will still take some of the pressure off your shoulders. And take the time to invest in other things outside of sport, but make sure they're things you actually enjoy doing.

It also must be said that everyone is different. What's right for me might not be right for you. We all look at life differently so don't judge yourself through someone else's lens. If you don't want to come back, or you don't feel up to it, that's okay as well.

SNOWBOARD CROSS

BELLE BROCKHOFF

Belle Brockhoff is an Australian snowboard cross athlete who has suffered two ACL ruptures to her right knee during her career. She underwent three surgeries—two reconstructions (utilising hamstring and patella grafts) and one 'clean out' arthroscope. Her rehabilitation was done in Australia. She has experienced competing both with and without her ACL.

I am a snowboard cross athlete and compete as part of the Australian national team on the World Cup Tour. Snowboard cross is similar to BMX racing, consisting of heats with four riders all racing down a course together, navigating obstacles such as jumps, rollers, turns and other varying features.

I've been to three Olympics so far—Sochi 2014, PyeongChang 2018, and Beijing 2022. I was climbing my way to the top of the world rankings, until my knee injuries slowed me down. I'm on the way back up again now after my second ACL reconstruction in 2018—finishing second in the world rankings at the end of my comeback season and becoming a World Champion in the team event—with Jarryd Hughes—the following season (2021). I was on the podium for World Cup events prior to the Beijing Olympics, however fell just short of a medal, finishing fourth at the Games.

I was lucky to have my Mum throw me into all kinds of sports from a young age. Tennis, soccer, football, cricket, softball, baseball, water polo, swimming—I really did a mix of everything. I also tried my hand at most winter sports—moguls, cross country skiing, and both alpine and freestyle skiing and snowboarding. But from the day I picked up my first snowboard at age 10, I knew I wanted to be one of the world's best snowboarders and to go to the Olympics. From 14 to 18, I focussed on alpine racing and giant slalom, but I wasn't getting the results I wanted. At 19, I switched to snowboard cross, and that's when the results started to come my way.

Many of my injuries over the years have come about from on- and off-snow training mishaps. When I was young, I definitely fell out of my fair share of trees. I also fell off the stage in my first interschools win! During training I've rolled my ankle badly in an agility session and had issues with tears in both of my quads during sprint training. You could argue snowboarders aren't made to be sprinters. My left wrist also has some problems after falling off a swiss ball! Not to mention quite a few concussions and a couple of KOs!

My first ACL happened in March 2017 at the Sierra Nevada (USA) World Championships. I was ranked number one in the world, was feeling amped up and really wanted to win my first world championship title. But I did my ACL before the competition even started.

I was selected to test the track, as I often had been that season. They choose a few top 10 riders to 'guinea pig' the course before training starts. But when I went to look at the track the day before, I felt a little nervous, which I'd never felt about testing before. That night I couldn't really figure out the flow of the course and its features in my mind. I couldn't remember anything.

When I dropped in for my test run, I remember being scared. I had such a lack of clarity in what I needed to do. I had tested many times before and had no issues with it but this time was for some reason, different. When I dropped into the track, I had no flow and crashed near the start section. I got up and rode down to the double, a feature that gives you no other option than to jump over two rollers. But for some reason I put the brakes on rather than keeping up my speed and tried to pump (ride) over them. I landed heavily on the up ramp of the second roller and my front knee (right) twisted before I was shot up into the air upside down due to the impact. I didn't feel a pop. Just a bit of soreness, and then it was fine. But when I stood up, I could feel my knee wasn't stable. Deep down I knew what I'd done, but I was hoping it was just a sprain.

I skipped official training the next day and had an MRI. I was still going through the motions believing I would be able to compete, but my body was telling me what I needed to know. During a pool session that day with our physio, I could feel my knee opening up sideways when I dragged it through the water. The MRI confirmed what I was feeling.

I cried for a second or two, before my rational side switched on. The Olympics were only 11 months away. I knew the recovery process of an ACL and how long it took to get back, so we came up with a plan straight away. I started my prehab the day after my MRI. I shifted gears really quickly, because I had to.

I flew home to have the surgery. I chose a hamstring graft because that was what my surgeon had most experience in and was comfortable using. It was what most people have, so I thought, 'Why not?' We did discuss using a cadaver graft, and my mum even put her hand up to give me her hamstring, but I didn't want to risk my body rejecting the graft with the Olympics so close, nor having my mum put her body through trauma. I didn't have time for anything to go wrong.

I was lucky it was an isolated ACL injury. In that case we didn't have to worry about cartilage healing timeframes and I could get straight into rehabbing in a serious way—seven days a week, five times a day. Rehab, ice, rehab, ice. My mum was a great help during the initial stages. In the mornings she would set up the Game Ready ice machine to do my first icing session before I'd even gotten out of bed. She was on a mission too.

I was also fortunate to have the great support of the Victorian Institute of Sport (VIS) for my rehab. With their help I returned to the snow quite quickly—at around four months during the Australian season. To be allowed to return to the snow, my right knee had to have at least 90 per cent of the strength of my left. I had to be able to do 50 single leg squats to 90 degrees, but since I'd had such an intense rehab, I managed to do 70-80 on each leg. My quads got so big I looked like a track cyclist! There were also hop tests, and a few others, and they were a good confidence test for me.

It was a careful return to snowboarding. I was wearing a custom knee brace, and only one lap was allowed at first, before I was gradually allowed to do more. Although we were pushing it with our timeframe before the Olympics, my strength and conditioning team, physio, and my coaches all worked well together.

I was ready to compete at around nine months, in December 2017, at the World Cup in Val Thorens in France. I had done everything to come back and be as strong as possible and I felt so strong and so ready. Physically I felt my knee could handle anything. Mentally, it was only because I hadn't had the chance to test out my knee racing yet that I wasn't quite 100 per cent confident.

At that first World Cup, I did my ACL again. My knee felt really good. I was riding well and I was riding fast. Conditions were perfect for our training days, and I was beating other girls in my heats who went on to make the podium at that World Cup. But on the day of our time trials, it started dumping snow. The visibility was appalling. It should have been cancelled. Quite a few athletes were injured—a few ACLs, a crushed ankle, a few concussions—more than usual. I was just one of them.

I dropped into the course and came undone over another double. This time I did jump over both rollers as I was meant to, but because the visibility was so bad, I mistimed my jump and landed with my legs fully extended rather than bent. As my right knee hyperextended, my ACL re-ruptured. I lay there and screamed with frustration. I knew immediately what had happened.

Our physio tested my knee almost immediately. He thought he could feel an endpoint, and I thought I could too. We were being optimistic. But in my heart, I knew that it was gone again. They did the test a few more times and then I just burst into tears on the table—one of the only times I've cried in front of my team. Not because I was in pain, more so because of all of the work I'd put in. I had been so disciplined and patient. And now to have another setback, with more damage to my knee (there was chondral cartilage and meniscus damage as well as bone bruising this time). And this being only two months out from the PyeongChang Olympics.

I processed things quickly again. While still on the table I said to my physio, 'I've still got to get to the Games.' I'd worked so hard for the last four years, I wasn't going to miss out. I didn't want to live with regrets, and I knew if I didn't try to make it to the Olympics, I'd regret it.

My only chance was to give it a shot without my ACL. I flew home, saw my same surgeon, and underwent a scope in late December to clean up the damaged cartilage and ACL. The best plan we had was to just rehab intensely after the scope and get as strong as possible so I could withstand the impacts needed for racing.

My rehab was similar to my ACL recovery, although I did all of my training in the gym wearing a knee brace. I was just trying to get the swelling down after surgery, and then training my knee to be stable and get the muscles firing. Lots of band, balance, and strength work.

I had already qualified for the Games, but still had to show I could perform for clearance by our medical team. The cut-off was for me to be able to compete at the Feldberg (Germany) World Cup in February, just before the Games. During that first event, it was the first time I had raced without an ACL and I didn't know how it would feel. There was still some bone bruising along with the cartilage damage, so riding was painful. Every impact hurt. Even just moving my leg up and down hurt.

But I managed to clock third fastest in time trials, and finish in eighth place, which gave me clearance to compete at the Olympics.

At PyeongChang the features were huge, much larger than what we were used to at the lead-up World Cups. For me it was struggle town. To ride, my knee had to be strapped with ridged tape and I wore a knee brace on top of that. The tape helped to make it feel more stable, but really restricted my movement—and in snowboard cross, particularly with larger features, you need full movement of your knees. The best I could managed with the tape was about 50 per cent of my normal range.

During the two training sessions (two days, two hours on each), I didn't make it fully down the track once. I crashed every time. I cut my face, injured my shoulder, and my snowboard binding exploded when I overshot one of the jumps because I couldn't bend my knee enough to fully compress. I'd never cracked a binding in my career. Things really weren't working in my favour. I don't usually watch my competitors, but I was watching that day. I only do that when I'm really lost. I wanted to see what they were doing to make it down the track, hoping it might help me figure out the best way I could get down the track. But all I was seeing was them get faster and faster and faster.

Come race day, I managed to complete just one lap down the course before the start of the time trials. I gave it everything I had with what I had to work with. I was basically on one leg, with no training laps! With each lap I started getting better and better, and I managed to make it through the rounds to the semi-final. From there, unfortunately I crashed towards the end of the course. Again, I just couldn't bend my knee fast enough for the jump, as I was getting faster with each lap. I finished 11th overall.

I remember crossing the finish line and collapsing to my knees and bursting into tears. It had been such a rollercoaster of emotions that had just been bottled up until I crossed that line. Because of the tight timeframe I had been on to get to the Games, I hadn't allowed myself to be sad, or mope around feeling sorry for myself. It was great to have made it that far, but all of the build-up of emotions finally came out at that moment.

Once the Olympics were over, I flew home and saw my same surgeon. Within a few weeks I underwent surgery again. As we'd already used my hamstring, we chose a quads tendon graft. The major difference this time around was that I had more time. We planned out my rehab, and when I could get back on the snow—this time it was at around six months, not four months as before. I wanted to take my time and give my knee the best possible chance, as much as I wanted to get out there. A great deal of patience was tested during this time.

Everything was on track and I snowboarded with the team at all of the overseas on-snow camps in December 2018. But I didn't compete. I was in no rush. I used the time to just get some on-snow mileage. That's what I did for the next year really. I didn't compete again until August 2019 at Mount Hotham—17 months after surgery.

Despite not racing, I continued training as best I could, and branched out into other sports. I picked up boxing again, which I had done before my knee injuries. And I also picked up training with an Australian rules footy player I was mentoring. She invited me to do a training session with her and an ex-AFL player and coach. I laced up my footy boots, and had fun doing lots of chopping and changing, jumping and landing, and quick reacting with the ball drills.

It was a great change from the plyometric and agility training in the gym that it is so controlled. It's great for some things, but there's often no reactive component to it. I found having someone else involved in the boxing and footy training, you have to react to that outside source. I think it definitely added extra percentages to my preparation. It was really different from what I had done the first time.

Leading up to my return season I was training really hard. I was pushing myself to challenge the boys as much as I could on snow—that pushed me to a level I wasn't used to. I always made sure that whatever training lap I did was with a guy who was faster than me; if I went by myself, I knew the intensity wouldn't be there due to my competitive nature.

My knee brace was with me again, but I found when I was wearing it

I would think about my knee negatively. I started riding without it, and soon decided not to wear it at all. Then I wasn't thinking about my knee anymore, and it was able to move in its natural way. I didn't wear a brace on my knee for the rest of the season.

When I returned to competing, my approach was to just see how it goes. I would aim for a few top 10 results. But after two years out of the sport I felt really ready to come back. I was sick of missing out on racing, so I was pretty fired up coming into the first World Cup in Montafon in Austria. I was able to stay calm, and in the moment, and it all just happened. In my first race back I came third, and I made the podium in five of the six World Cups that season. I also finished up as world number two, just shy of number one.

The big thing that changed for me was not the physical aspect, but my mental game. I'd come back a lot stronger mentally. Patience, being calm, and thinking with more clarity was now part of my racing. That continued into the next season where I won the 2021 World Championship gold in the mixed team event at Idre (Sweden) with Jarryd Hughes—who has also had his fair share of knee issues with five left knee surgeries. Between us we've had eight knee surgeries!

My knee is no longer an issue. Although I didn't get the result I would have liked at Beijing, I still feel I have many years of racing left in me. And I'm hungrier than ever to win.

REFLECTIONS

My ACL journeys were far from perfect. Yet despite the obvious setbacks at the time, I am happy I went through it all. I would still take my knee injuries any day because I've learned so much from them.

One of the main factors that lead to me injuring my ACL the first time

was that I let the emotion of fear come in. I was nervous and scared about the track testing that day but felt like I needed to prove to people that I was fearless and great. Although I knew I had to jump the rollers, my clarity of thought and decision-making just went out the window. I should have pulled out, but I didn't. I'm smarter than that now.

I suspect my ACL had been tearing gradually over a number of years from the hard life I was putting it through. I'd had a number of incidences where I'd had flat landings or crashed into fences and had pain for a couple of days, but it would always settle.

The poor conditions contributed to my second ACL. Soon after I was injured, they cancelled the day's racing. In hindsight all of the riders should have stood up collectively and said it was too dangerous. We should have refused to race, and had the time trials postponed. I'm not afraid these days to tell race organisers what I think. But you need the collective voice to make changes, not just one opinion. Some of the time many riders do feel pressured to have to compete no matter what, and we have the responsibility to voice this. Ultimately though, I do think that I was mostly just plain unlucky when I re-ruptured my ACL. It could have happened to any rider. I don't think I was under-prepared. I felt good and strong.

I was fortunate to be given ACL advice by fellow winter athletes I respected who had been through their own injury journeys. Before the Games, French snowboard cross athlete Pierre Vaultier pretty much gave me a roadmap of what I needed to do. He's considered by many to be the GOAT of our sport, having won two Olympic gold medals and more than 30 World Cups and Crystal Globes. I felt anything he said would be good advice. My teammate Jarryd Hughes, who despite his own knee issues has still managed to win X Games gold, Olympic silver, and our recent team World Championship gold, also shared some wisdom. He told me, 'Don't be a hero' by returning too soon. Lydia Lassila, Australian aerial skiing Olympic Champion who also has overcome knee injuries, also reached out. Fellow Australian aerial skiing champion Jacqui Cooper has supported me during my journey and still does!

Knowing other winter athletes who had injured their ACLs meant I already had some idea about what was involved. Things like graft choice, and the rehab process. They also told me what it would be like mentally but it's one thing to be told vs actually going through it. You get thrown in the deep end with that side of things. It was challenging.

Mentally I found the things that help me most were 'doing' things rather than talking. The boxing and footy training really helped, as both involved being completely present and focused. I also started playing Mario Kart (a Nintendo game) while cycling at home, with the idea being to increase my focus threshold under fatigue. You're sweating, breathing heavily, all while playing Mario and focussing on racing. I feel that combining my concentration and racing skills with fatigue elements really helped my mental game.

If I had to pinpoint an aspect of my rehab that didn't go well, it was the clarity surrounding my return-to-snow plan. Although the team around me was great, the system around the return-to-sport process during my first ACL wasn't. It wasn't made clear to me what exactly I had to do to get back on the snow. Every time I passed what I thought was the final test, the goalposts would be moved. It was a constant rollercoaster of emotions and had more effect on me emotionally than actually being stuck in rehab. All I wanted was to be given a checklist of what I needed to do. One did exist, it was just that I hadn't been shown it. There was a definite lack of communication between all parties in that instance. That wasn't an issue the second time around. I believe my feedback may have improved things from then on.

As for what went well, it was the learning curve of the whole experience— it changed me as a person. I'm now able to see myself and my sport differently. When I returned to competing, I was nervous about racing with riders around me again. But I was fine. I was more than fine. For the first time ever, I was able to battle my way through the heats. Even if I was coming last, I was able to work my way around the girls to win every heat and progress to the next round. I made the big final every single time in that 2019/20 season. And during the racing I was incredibly calm, which I'd never experienced before. It was a totally new thing for me.

I also learned how incredible my body can be—both with healing, and with adapting to what I need to put it through to keep getting stronger and improving. I realised quickly that I had to keep my training up. If I didn't, my muscles would deflate and my leg would become a noodle very quickly! It sounds simple, but I know now how important it is to take care of my body.

As I'm getting older, I've noticed more and more that I just need to take that little bit of extra care in recovery, and with what I'm putting into my body. I go gluten-free in competition week and during heavy training. I love bread and carbs, but I know that if I have gluten my knee gets really swollen and sore. If I don't have gluten, I don't have any of the symptoms from my injury. I am open to experimenting with a lot of things, and as a result have become much more in tune with my body.

My injuries have also helped me to become more patient. I still have a long way to go, but they really made me step back. I was always GO! GO! GO! before. I felt I had to become the best, to get results on top of results to secure funding and sponsors. I'd be the first girl to drop in the gates because I didn't want to be seen as a wimp. But now, I'm happy to watch everyone else go first. I get to relax and watch. If I miss out on one practice run because of it, then so be it. That was how I approached things during my return season, and it worked for me.

Before my ACL injuries I didn't formally track my periods, although I roughly knew my cycle. Each time I've done my ACL I was on the second or third day of my period, and I do feel my cycle most likely contributed to my injuries. I get really bad period pain and don't feel very switched on when I am on my period. My energy levels drop, my clarity is down, and I'm in pain. It's not ideal for performing well! I am aware that our ligaments become laxer at certain times in the cycle, and that our coordination can be altered when we're on our period. But it is only recently that trainers have started to consider these changes and talk about it with regard to my training. I'm glad I have an open-minded trainer who can cater to these cycles when I have them.

Only recently do I now take the pill. The main reason being so I can manipulate my cycle, as managing your period on top of a mountain for a whole day of racing can be challenging! I skip my periods during the competition season, then return to a normal cycle once I get back home.

One of the things that helped me to push through without an ACL for the PyeongChang Olympics was the fact that I'd seen other athletes in my sport do amazing things without an ACL. Pierre Vaultier, whom I mentioned earlier, won at the Sochi Olympics without an ACL. He had the exact timeframe as me—he tore it two months out, did intensive rehab, and came back and won gold. I just thought, 'Why can I not do that too? I can totally do it'. It's just having the will to do it.

It did take me a while to stop worrying about my knee when I was snowboarding without my ACL. But I had so much tape I didn't really feel any instability. During my gym sessions it felt fine. Occasionally it felt a bit loose with certain movements, but I felt that as I got stronger things kept improving. I had no collapsing or anything like that.

I did consider not repairing my knee after the Olympics. I was aware of others coming back to sport within the year successfully without an ACL. But I didn't really know all that much about it. It seemed like a new sort of area that people are starting to look into and consider, that you may not need an ACL, that it might grow back. But I didn't want to wait or have any uncertainty, so I chose to do the surgery and the rehab again and come back that way. I just wanted to get back to my best possible form without any doubts in my mind.

I did change my approach to how quickly I returned to competing. I had previously thought that the standard ACL recovery time was around nine to 12 months. But I was hearing people say that true recovery was more like 24 months. I could have come back in a year, but felt like I would prefer to gain the extra percentage of risk reduction that the research shows you get where you don't compete in your sport too soon. For me, it was around the 16- to 17-month mark when I felt a huge shift in my body and the way it functioned.

If I had to give advice to my younger self, it would be to slow down. What's the rush in getting results so fast? Although I thought I gained so much knowledge with that full-steam-ahead approach initially, I totally lacked any awareness and experience. Patience is a virtue.

My advice to others who have done their ACL would be to respect and be aware of the return-to-sport process. And take your time. If you really want to come back, do the rehab properly and don't skip sessions. If you don't do the rehab, you're going to be worse off. But to *really* come back better than before, you have to do more than just the prescribed rehab. It will give you your foundations, but you have to think outside the box to find those extra one-percenters.

RUGBY UNION

DAMIEN FITZPATRICK

Damien Fitzpatrick is a professional rugby player who underwent five left-knee surgeries during his Australian and international career—two arthroscopic surgeries for cartilage damage followed by a string of three ACL ruptures in 18 months. His first four surgeries and rehabilitations took place in Australia, while his final surgery (after a third ACL reconstruction) and recovery were undertaken in France. Both hamstring and patella grafts were utilised for his ACL reconstructions, with his third also including a tibial osteotomy.

I played rugby union in the front row as a hooker. I made my Super Rugby debut for the New South Wales (NSW) Waratahs in 2009 aged 19, so I had a professional rugby career now spanning over 12 years. In that time, I played for three professional sides—the Waratahs in Australia, and Lyon and *Stade Français* in the French National Rugby League Top 14. My main team throughout the years has been the Waratahs, which, for a Sydney-born and raised kid, has been a dream come true. To have the opportunity to represent the team I grew up supporting has been amazing.

I played a lot of sport as a kid. I had asthma growing up so my parents put me into swimming early and I loved it. I did a lot of squad and competitive swimming all through school, and I've continued to swim all through my rugby career. I also played basketball and tennis, but swimming and rugby were the two main sports for me. I went through the ranks with my junior rugby career playing at state level and captained the Australian Schoolboys side at 18. I followed that up in 2009 by captaining the under 20s, before making my debut in Super Rugby that same year.

Injuries haven't been kind to me over the years. In year 12 I broke four bones in my hand, and in my first year out of school playing senior club rugby I dislocated my wrist. I remember looking down seeing my arm bent at a right angle—it was quite the experience. I've also had surgery on a broken scaphoid, torn the PCL in my right knee, and broken my sternum, a rib and my clavicle.

My first major left knee injury came when I was 15. I had an arthroscope to remove a large chunk of cartilage that had come off the back of my patella from the impact of someone's head colliding against my knee as we dived for a ball. I went from a few weeks on crutches, to running again at around six weeks with minimal rehab or activation exercises. To say my left knee has since been my problem knee is somewhat of an understatement!

At 21, I injured my left knee again. It was my second season playing for the Waratahs and I was super keen to do anything that my teammates asked of me. One of the very influential players (Drew Mitchell) asked me to kick and catch some high balls with him. I went to leap in the air and catch the ball but came down on my left knee at a poor angle and heard a massive crack. I knew immediately something wasn't right but was pretty embarrassed and tried not to show that I'd injured myself. I kept saying I was okay, and tried to complete my training, but I quickly realised my knee was not right. The team doctor caught wind of what was going on and suggested we get a scan. I think she probably knew something was wrong.

I'd torn my medial meniscus completely in half. A piece had bent itself back and jammed inside my knee. The idea was to try to sew it back together, but unfortunately that couldn't happen, and I underwent another arthroscope to remove the flap (medial meniscectomy).

At six weeks after the surgery I was right to start a very modified running program. But I went against excellent medical advice and tried to rush back—something I've been guilty of a few times in my career. Although there was no pressure on me to return to play, I started doing things on the sly and pretty much went from zero to match-style running. Within about a week I'd created a stress fracture on the top of my tibia, and needed another 12 weeks off the field. If I'd just waited another few weeks!

For the remainder of 2011 I went back and played club rugby. We had a great season and ended up winning the grand final. Riding that high, I went into 2012 preseason feeling really strong and fit and thinking the season ahead was going to be a great one. I was the only player to complete every single minute of every session that preseason. I was turning 22, and it was the perfect time for me to stamp my claim at belonging at the professional level. Unfortunately, that wasn't to be.

I did my first ACL in round three. I came off the bench and was running around and everything felt okay. I tracked across the field in defence and my opponent did a slight stutter step. I jammed my foot down to react to the way he was moving, and my foot caught in the ground. My left knee moved in a really peculiar way and I heard a massive pop. I fell over myself, and my opponent fell on top of me making it look like I'd tackled him. But it was my knee buckling that put me on the ground, not the contact.

I remember thinking I'd never been in so much pain in my entire life. I ended up at the bottom of a ruck, which is when a lot of players pile up on top of one another. I couldn't get out so kept yelling, 'Watch my leg!' as I grabbed my knee and tried to move away. I knew something wasn't right. It was like nothing was holding my knee together—it felt so unstable. I didn't get up and try to run or play on, I stayed on the ground until the whistle blew and our doctor was able to come out and assess me.

I didn't know what I'd done. I knew what an ACL injury was, and knew a few people who'd had that injury, but it didn't spring to mind immediately as to what I had done. Our usual doctor wasn't with us that game, and it was her stand-in's first night on the job. He ran on and was very professional, and did the Lachman's test, but was unable to hide what he was assessing. I could tell straight away from his face that something wasn't right. That was quickly confirmed when he spoke on the radio saying, 'He's not going to be right to play on,' followed by his response to the coach's query as to why: 'He's done his ACL'.

I was taken straight into the changerooms and immediately started icing my knee. The team won, so it was a bittersweet atmosphere. The boys all came in at the end celebrating, but many of them came over to me asking if I was all right. The doc sent me home with the Game Ready unit and I pretty much stayed up the entire night icing and compressing my knee to reduce the swelling before we flew back to Sydney from Melbourne the next morning. I had an MRI that showed a tear to my ACL but with no cartilage damage. I was booked in for surgery two days later.

We chose to do the surgery straight away. It was the beginning of the season and there was still rugby to be played later in the year. My knee was still pretty blown up with quite a bit of swelling. From what I remember there wasn't really a discussion about different graft types, it was more presented to me as, 'This is what we're doing'. We used a hamstring graft as I think it was the surgeon's preferred method, and our doc was comfortable with it as other Waratah players had also had the same graft. I was happy to go along with whatever was suggested. No conservative option was discussed. The conversation was pretty much, 'This is what's happened, this is what we need to do about it, let's do it'.

I completed around 10 months of very thorough inhouse rehab with the Waratahs. We did a lot of leg strengthening and muscular endurance exercises, VMO work—all of that kind of stuff. That was mirrored with a pretty extensive running and return-to-play sequence of ball retrievals, and reactionary and non-reactionary change of direction work. There wasn't a movement I was going to be exposed to on the field that I hadn't done in my rehab.

I never got back to playing to test it out. On the first day I was given the green light to start training fully with the team, I ended up tearing my ACL again halfway through the session. I was a little bit nervous on returning to full training. We had a new coach and I think there was some anxiety to get everyone right and back on the field. I did some warmup drills with the team, and then we were lined up for the yoyo (beep) test. I remember the coach asking the strength and conditioning coach if I was right to do it, and the coach said he didn't see why not because I'd done the movements we were about to do, and under fatigued conditions, so he didn't think it would be any different. Unfortunately, it was.

I got up to level 16.2. As I hit the 20-metre interval line to turn around, I just felt this slight click in my knee. More like the small pop you get when you click your finger joints. It was nothing like the first time. It was really odd. Again, there was no contact. And my foot didn't slip. But I hit the ground and stayed down while everyone else kept running. The pain was almost non-existent. I thought I was okay, even though I was rubbing the back of my knee a little. I was able to stand up and walk off. It didn't feel unstable.

The physio ran over and did the usual tests. He had this very strange look on his face when he did the Lachman's test, and even I could feel that there wasn't any stop to the movement. I thought, 'Oh no, this isn't good'. He was very experienced and conscious of where my head would be at having redone my ACL on my first day back in training. He just said, 'I think that will do you for the day. Why don't you go down and see the doc and touch base?' I'm sure he knew exactly what had happened but didn't want to make the call on the field.

By the time I reached our doctor, she had already received a call from the physio so knew exactly what was going on. She took me into her office and went through all of the tests again, also with a strange look on her face. I think the words she used were, 'That's really bizarre, what you're telling me doesn't match up with what I'm feeling. It's probably best we get a scan.' Our radiographer was right next door, so almost immediately we got an MRI and realised I had done my ACL again, and just doing something so innocuous.

I was pretty shattered when we got the results. Because of the way the season was aligned I had chosen to continue my rehab and train through my annual leave in October. After that day of pre-season training and testing I was booked to go on a well-needed holiday to Hawaii, with my girlfriend. I remember closing the blinds in our doc's office and saying, 'This is going to be really tough for me to take. I don't want tell my parents yet as they worry more than I do. I don't even want my girlfriend to know. I just want to go on holidays before dealing with my knee'. She agreed I needed a break and time away to process things and thought Hawaii would be good for me mentally. But she did suggest I should tell people.

So the holiday went ahead, but I managed not to talk to anyone, not even my girlfriend, about my injury. It was a strange time. When I was walking on the beach there were definitely a few episodes of instability, but I would try to hide it as I didn't want to ruin our trip. I also remember running on the treadmill in the hotel gym and my knee feeling fine. I did eventually tell my girlfriend just before we came back, and by the time we arrived home I was ready to face the music. I knew I wasn't going to be playing any time soon—I was ready to go in for another surgery.

We did another scan just to double check everything, and then I went back to see the same surgeon. We talked about the fact that re-ruptures do occur and went over everything. We were trying to work out if there was anything we could have done differently. That's when we really focussed in on the graft. We were wondering whether there may have been something there that was the issue. We looked at some of the earlier MRIs, and at around the six-month mark it showed the graft was not quite as bold and black as it should have been, a tell-tale sign the graft hadn't taken as well as it should have. We mostly discussed how we were trying to fix the issue and what the next surgery would look like. It was decided that obviously

I had quite a lax joint and that a tighter graft might be an option, so we chose to do a patella tendon graft. Again, a conservative option was never discussed, more so that we just needed to get some stability into the joint. With me being only 22, they knew there was some time on my side in terms of my career, so the benefits of trying to stabilise my joint as much as possible was considered the best option.

Compared to my first ACL, this time around I walked into surgery almost feeling like I could play. It didn't feel unstable like the first one. I'd say that was partially to do with how much rehab I'd already done. My legs were so muscly and solid at the time. It hadn't swollen that much either, and whatever there was went down very quickly and had gone before the surgery.

There was more focus the second time around on my mental health. All I'd really had in terms of a break between the first failed ACL rehab and the start of the second was that two-week holiday in Hawaii. I had the same rehab team working with me and everyone was aware it was going to become long and laborious for me quite quickly, so they were flexible and proactive in helping me get through that. The medical staff knew I loved swimming, so they incorporated it into my rehab. In the mornings I would tick off my cardio work with a swimming squad, and in the afternoons I would complete my main rehab. With quite a bit of residual strength left over from the first rehab, we did more balance and stability work this time and less focus on just absolute strength and volume.

My rehab was around 10 months again. By the time I returned to playing in July it was the end of the season. I felt like I needed a change after having been injured for two full years and was really eager to play. The European season started in August, whereas the Australian season wasn't until February, so I signed a contract with Lyon in France so I could play almost immediately.

My girlfriend and I relocated to France. I got back on the field and everything was feeling really good. I was playing well. I did around a month of training, and played eight games when again, a very similar, very innocuous thing occurred. I was running laterally following the defence along the field and I just squared up in front my opponent to make the tackle and did a little bit of footwork. My knee got in a funny position and again, I just felt a little 'click'. I thought nothing of it and continued to play and keep running. It was nearly the end of the game and I'd played a lot of minutes, and I started rubbing my knee. The physio came running on, and with only 10 minutes left they were happy to make the substitution. I went off the field and told the coach that everything was okay.

That night everything still seemed fine. I had not even considered it would be my ACL. I thought maybe I'd done a bit of cartilage damage. I had a little bit of pain behind my knee, but nothing that I thought would have meant I would have done my ACL again. The French are very conservative with injury—they will scan almost everything. So even though I was saying very loudly that I didn't need a scan, the next morning after seeing the doctor—who again had the strange look on his face when he tested my knee—I had an MRI that unfortunately showed I'd ruptured my graft again. I couldn't believe it.

I was speechless. I thought it was all just hopeless. Quite a few dark thoughts started to come into my mind. The doctor was a very caring man, but he just said, 'You've got a decision to make—let us know what you're thinking'. I spoke to my parents who gently suggested, 'Your body is telling you it shouldn't play rugby anymore. It's time to do something else'. I was starting to think that way as well. It was a shame. My girlfriend and I had just moved over to France and started a new life, but the decision looked like it was going have to be that I stop playing.

Then I got called back into the club. They said, 'You're 24. You've had three ACLs in 18 months. And you've only been back on the field for two months. Something doesn't add up here. Before you make the decision to retire, would you consider seeing a specialist here in Lyon?' I asked what the point was, thinking there would be no difference from the specialists I'd already seen. The doctor gave me the specialist's name and told me to Google him. It turned out he conducted conferences all over the world and his reputation seemed as impressive as they had said. When I mentioned him to some of the French players, they all praised him as Europe's best knee surgeon. He was also a big fan of rugby and happy to fit me in. I figured I had nothing to lose, so I went and saw him the next morning.

He was an eccentric bloke in a big white coat with two or three helpers in his room. I couldn't really speak French at that point, but luckily he spoke English—although he had barely looked at me when I first entered his room. He just handed me a wad of papers for all of the different scans he wanted. Apparently when he'd heard my story, he thought there was something being missed. He sent me for bone density scans, another MRI, and more x-rays. But one of the x-rays was from side on; he wanted to compare the angle of my tibial slope from one leg to the other. I had never heard of that before.

When I went back to see him, I handed him a massive pile of scans. He threw them all onto the table, except the one showing the tibial slope comparison. He looked at the x-rays briefly and exclaimed, 'Voila!' It was exactly what he thought the problem would be. The tibial slope on my left leg was 15 degrees, and my right was eight degrees. He went on to explain, 'Imagine your left ACL is like a guitar string, we have to move it from the left side of your femur to the right side of your tibia, but with your knee that's too far for it to move. So, every time we do an ACL reconstruction on you, it will be too tight, and any slight movement will cause the ACL to snap. Right now, with your leg like this, there's no hope for you to continue playing professional sport.' I thought, 'Ok, at least we know why now.' But he said, 'I think I can fix it.' He'd seen this issue before on two professional soccer players in Europe and had fixed the problem.

When I asked how, he replied, 'Grande surgery.' I knew enough French to know what that meant. It would require a tibial osteotomy—he would cut a wedge out of my tibia to take the slope angle back to the eight degrees it was on the right. At the same time, he would reconstruct my ACL again, but for extra stability would include a Macintosh Loop— using a piece of my ITB to reinforce the outside of my knee. He said, 'If you're willing to do this, I could get it done. And you'll be the only rugby player in the world to have it done.' His parting words were, 'Think about it, and talk to your club. If you'd like to go ahead, we can book it in and get it sorted.'

The club was supportive of whatever I decided. My parents thought it sounded like too big an operation and that it was perhaps time to finish up, and my girlfriend said it was my decision. I felt I really only had one more shot at this, and if I'd found a surgeon who thought he could have a go at it, I'd be silly not to try. Once I'd decided to do it, I didn't really put too much further thought into the surgery, but I probably should have. I didn't look into what an osteotomy actually meant—essentially that your leg is going to be broken, how long the surgery would be (five hours), or how big the recovery would be (long).

Four other surgeons flew in from South America to watch. When I woke up to strange men speaking Spanish, they all told me he had performed a 'beautiful surgery'. But when I looked down at my left leg it was covered from my ankle to my groin with bandages, and both of my legs were elevated as he'd used a patella graft from my right side. The surgeon said he was happy with the surgery, but when the bandages came off the bruising was spectacular. It went all the way up and down my leg. Looking down for the first time, I wondered what had the surgeon done—had I let him butcher my leg? Compared to the usual small cuts from a standard ACL surgery, there was a big one on the side of my leg because of the Macintosh Loop, and a huge cut down the front for the osteotomy. It looked like something out of Frankenstein.

I don't think I've ever been in more pain in my life. I discovered that bones hurt, a lot. After around a week in the Lyon hospital I was moved to a recovery facility for a further three weeks. There they slowly got me doing some basic physio, which was a painful change after spending two weeks in a wheelchair with two straight knees. It was like I was recovering from a major trauma surgery, and I guess I was in a way.

Playing rugby again seemed a million miles away. I couldn't even consider playing professional sport again. I was meant to spend another two weeks in the rehab centre but I hated it so much I complained to the team that if they didn't get me out, I was going to let myself out. They convinced the rehab centre to let me go home in a wheelchair. I remember my girlfriend pushing me around in Lyon—which is full of cobblestoned streets—with my leg out straight. I learned quickly that cobble stones and wheelchairs don't mix!

The rehab was different from the others. The initial focus was on not damaging the leg any further. The bone needed to heal so it was a good six weeks of doing not much aside from keeping my leg straight, and then another six weeks of gently starting to get it moving. It wasn't until the 12 to 15 weeks mark that rehab started to get going. There was definitely more control and balance work than I'd done previously, less focus on absolute strength again, and more on body weight strength and single leg work. There was also a lot more use of ultrasound, electrotherapy gadgets, and techniques like scar-scraping to help break down scar tissue to improve my knee's mobility.

We pushed things a little too far at one stage and I started getting quite a bit of pain. I ended up having another tibial stress fracture where my patella tendon had been cut and flipped back during the osteotomy. The stress fracture was so bad it needed another surgery, so they replaced it with a section of bone grafted from my hip and secured it with a bracket over the top. That set me back for another two months.

Overall it was just over 12 months until I was able to return to playing. The surgeon would have known how long it would take, but no one told me it would be that long. He had the final say on everything. I think one of the reasons he was so keen to take me on was to have the claim for being the first surgeon to put a rugby player back on the field with a tibial osteotomy. But that would only work if I made it back successfully. So, he was very conservative every step of the way, especially after the stress fracture incident. I would get to the next stage in my rehab, be cleared by the team doctor to progress, then I'd go to the surgeon and he'd say, 'No'. That happened two or three times. But it was exactly what I needed.

When I did return, I felt like I was made of glass for around six weeks. Mentally it took a long time to really feel confident in my knee again, and it's never really gone back to feeling 100 per cent. I would say that mentally I'm always at around 80 per cent with that knee. Although I have been able to get back and play competitively again, there's always that something in the back of my mind after all my knee has gone through. I'm limited in my training as to how much weight I can lift, so all of my metrics show it's a weakened knee. But when you see my scans it's understandable as there's a hefty amount of metal in there, combined with the amount of cartilage I'm missing.

These days it's the arthritis that causes me the most problems. I think this stems from having had significant cartilage loss behind my patella and on the medial side from such a young age. As well as the instability caused by the number of reconstructions. I only have anterior knee pain from my patella grafts when I'm kneeling, but it has hurt when going downstairs since my early 20s.

I find my VMO switches off really easily and I have trouble with my catch landings and that sort of thing. Before any training or games, I make sure I've thoroughly rolled out the leg and done a bunch of activation work on steps of different heights. I've also started a new jumping warmup I complete with one of the physios right before we hit the field on a blow-up mat. During weights I do a lot of banded work on my knee. Lots of lateral squats with bands and pulling the knee in different directions with a small focus around that VMO to make sure I can keep it firing as best as possible.

Unfortunately, my knee is a bit of a ticking timebomb for me, but it is what it is. The surgeon in Lyon was able to get another four or five years of professional rugby out of me and I'm grateful to have been given the opportunity to play again. Without his input I would have had to retire at 24 and fallen into the 'what could have been' category.

It had always been a dream of mine to play for the Wallabies. I feel I was on the right path until my ACL issues lead to three years out of the game.

While I haven't reached the career heights I had hoped, I've learned to cope with what I've been dealt and go along a different path.

REFLECTIONS

Despite the setbacks and hardship my knee has caused, there's not much I would change. The first time everyone was telling me I was young and not the first 22-year-old to have an ACL injury playing professional rugby. They were saying, 'You'll be back stronger. The months will fly by. Use the time to improve other parts of your body.' There was nothing I could fault in the rehab process. I did everything by the book, and it was perhaps just the graft that let me down. My only question would be around why we didn't pick that up earlier on the scans.

I knew the second time around was going to be very different. I was lucky our team doctor was so aware of my state of mind and took account of me as a person. She kept a very close watch on how I was reacting and organised extra help from a sports psychologist—not because I was immediately struggling, but more as a preventative thing. I was open to it for a few sessions and learned some really good coping mechanisms to help me deal with what I was facing. Having to go through the whole rehab process again without having stepped back on the field, and the fact returning to play was all so close before the goalposts moved on me.

I enjoyed being part of the team environment while I completed my first rehab. I could still be around the boys and joke about things. But the second year I found it hard to be around the group when they were training. It made me feel more distant and upset, so we organised my rehab schedule so that I did squad swimming early in the morning, some work experience in the middle of the day, and then training at the club once the guys had gone home. That way I didn't have to watch them on the field.

Completing a really good session of squad swimming and being part of a

different team environment was exactly what I needed to get me through the second rehab. Being able to really exert myself physically in the pool also helped me to release some of my frustrations and make me feel as though I was achieving something again, even though I wasn't able to achieve what I wanted on the field.

As for the third ACL, I was just amazed and frustrated at why that difference of the tibial slope angle hadn't been picked up in Australia. I was a bit annoyed I'd had to find out in France. But I realise we all live in our little bubbles around the world and think we have the best systems and practices—and there are always the outliers. Unfortunately, that was me.

In France at least everything was new and exciting. If I was still in Sydney during that third rehab, it would have been incredibly hard. Having never been to Europe before, once I got through the difficult initial healing stage and went back to the team to start my rehab, the fact I was in such a foreign country cast everything in a new light. When I wasn't rehabbing, we were out exploring France. We loved living in the city of Lyon. And I was practising my French. I was trying to immerse myself in the culture and I think that really helped. It wasn't like at home where I'd walk down the street and see people I knew and have the same conversations: 'How's your injury going? How are you feeling? When are you back?' I was out of the bubble and able to concentrate on life outside of rehab and rugby.

I never got down on myself for being injured. That was one thing I was lucky with. While there were tough days, I always felt that if I trained hard enough, I could get back to where I needed to be. That was one way I always coped with it all.

I knew I was resilient, but I did surprise myself with how I just kept bouncing back. I was able to keep training and not get bored doing it. I realised I didn't mind routine, and I didn't mind doing something over and over again, particularly when it came to training. I know other athletes can struggle with it—the motivation to keep training and keep going—but I didn't have any moments like that.

I've often thought about how these types of challenges can change you as a person. One of the biggest changes for me was moving to France—I don't think I would have gone there if it wasn't for my injuries. The three years we were living there away from family and friends changed my whole perception of the world, and I think for the better. It opened my eyes to a love of so many other things outside of rugby that I didn't even know existed. It also accelerated my preparation for life outside of sport.

Until my second ACL I was very focused on rugby. I was doing university at the time too but wasn't in any rush to complete my degree. After my third ACL I realised that life after rugby was coming much sooner for me than I first thought. I knew from that moment that if I was able to get back on the field, I would make a plan and be sure I was prepared for when rugby ended. I was lucky to continue playing but was aware that it could all get taken away from me quickly. My injuries definitely made me prepared for what was to come after sport, and probably a little more comfortable with the thought of retirement than other athletes.

If I had my time again, I would probably take a more conservative approach on a lot of things. There was something in my head that said if I could do more than was asked it would prove that I would be right to play earlier. I always pushed it harder than I needed to. I've always taken that mindset into my training, but it wasn't the right one for my rehabs. It took me a while to realise that, and it's something that I definitely regret now. There are rewards for people who are able to complete their rehab well, but there are no rewards for completing just the first piece of rehab well, so you may as well take your time through it.

If I could give my younger self some advice, I would say be patient. Don't feel that everything has to come at once. Listen to your medical advice and make sure you can take some extra weeks if possible. It's really not worth the extra damage you could do and potential games you might miss to try to hurry through any stage of your rehab. My advice to others would be even if you're feeling good, try to tell yourself it doesn't feel as good as you think. Take 10 per cent off. If you feel like you're at 80 per cent, tell yourself you're only at 70 per cent. Just wait a little bit longer. There's nothing wrong with being a bit more conservative.

Stay positive. Things are going to become routine, and become a process that you've got to do, so just stay positive with it. Try to seek some outcomes each week so you can work through them, and at the end of each week you can see progression and feel like you've achieved something.

CRICKET

CALLUM FERGUSON

Callum Ferguson is an Australian professional cricketer who sustained three ACL injuries during his career—one partial tear and one full rupture to his right knee, and a full rupture of his left. He underwent surgery for all three injuries in Australia, requiring only a 'clean out' for his partial tear, while hamstring grafts were utilised for each of his subsequent full reconstructions. His three rehabilitation periods were all completed in Australia.

I am a professional Australian cricketer who has represented Australia in all three forms of international cricket. In 2021 I retired from first-class cricket with the South Australian Redbacks in Australia's Sheffield Shield and one-day domestic competitions. I also stepped away from the Big Bash League, after I had captained the Sydney Thunder and played for the Adelaide Strikers and Melbourne Renegades.

I have been lucky to have had a long career. I had previously played for Worcestershire in the Rapids T20 competition, and the Pune Warriors in the Indian Premier League. My first rookie contract with the South Australian (SA) Redbacks was at 16, and I made my debut at 18. Now more than 20 years later, I've been in the system for a long time. I am unsure if I will play again. I have enjoyed this summer working in the media. I am keeping myself in shape while I decide.

I come from a tennis family, so was a bit of a black sheep for playing cricket. My father was a professional tennis player for a short period, and my mother was a number-one State League tennis player in South Australia. My brother also played tennis in the junior grand slams and professionally on tour before he went to university on a tennis scholarship. His career was cut short due to cartilage damage in both knees. Mum also had a knee reconstruction in her mid-twenties. Some might suggest there's a genetic link, as historically knees have been a problem within our family!

Sport was a huge part of my growing up. As well as tennis, I was also playing Australian rules football. But I remember saying to Dad one night that I'd decided I wanted to really have a crack at cricket. It was quite young to be deciding which career path to take, but that was the decision I made, and I haven't regretted it one bit. Through my cricket career, I've been fortunate to have only missed 10 games or so due to injuries other than my ACLs. I've had a pretty charmed run, aside from my knees.

My first ACL injury was in 2004. It was during the last warm-up game before the Under 19 World Cup in Bangladesh. I was 18. I was batting and running between the wickets for a second run. For some reason my partner had swapped sides, meaning we were running on the same side of the wicket. In trying to avoid him, I moved to my left, but as I went to push off my right knee gave way. I felt a tearing sensation. It wasn't so much the 'pop' a lot of people talk about, more of a tear. I fell forward and knew something was wrong straight away. But I still managed to crawl to my crease to make sure I didn't get run out! Even when injured your mind is always on the game!

The physio came out and removed my pad to do basic knee tests. He didn't give too much away, but as I walked off the ground, I could feel my knee was a little unstable. It was quite painful initially, and then it went numb. The physio again had a good look once we made it to the changerooms. I could tell he wasn't overly confident in my knee. When I went back to my teammates and was talking them through what had happened, I started to feel nauseous and vomited. I think it was all part of the shock of it all. That was definitely me done for the day.

After the game we went to a hospital. Sitting in the waiting room was quite an experience. It was the busiest hospital I had ever seen. Thankfully they got me into an MRI relatively quickly. The doctor came to our hotel that evening and told me it all looked pretty good. He showed me my scans—where the ACL and PCL were still crossing over—and said I should be okay in about 10 days. We all looked at each other thinking, 'Wow, that wasn't what we were expecting.' My knee was the size of a basketball.

I spent the next few days quite unwell. I had picked up a stomach bug, which made getting up and down from my bed to the bathroom with a sore knee pretty difficult. My stomach soon got better, but after a week or so my knee still wasn't showing any signs of improvement. I was put on a plane home not long after.

The first surgeon I saw took one look at my knee and said, 'You're going to need a full reconstruction.' It was an interesting consultation. He seemed very blasé about it all and wasn't at all personable. It was already a tough scenario to take at that age and having made my debut for South Australia in the previous season, it felt like my world was crumbling down. Not feeling very comfortable about that first appointment didn't help.

My aunt is a nurse and suggested I seek a second opinion. She knew an orthopaedic surgeon who looked after a lot of footballers in South Australia and had a really good reputation, so I went and saw him. He was much more personable and seemed to understand it was quite a stressful time and reassured me. He ordered another MRI which contradicted the original one taken in Bangladesh and explained that although there was a real possibility he would need to do a full reconstruction, until he 'went in' he couldn't be 100 per cent sure.

He was able to get me in quickly. I went into surgery expecting the worst. But when I woke up, he gave me the news that I hadn't needed a full reconstruction. I still had 70 per cent of my natural-born ACL functioning and he believed that would be as strong if not stronger than a graft. He had tidied up my damaged ACL and repaired the meniscus as best he could. The repair meant my rehab was extended to five months, rather than a shorter period if it had just been a standard clean out. It was still significantly less than the full ACL rehab I was expecting. That great news combined with the drugs from surgery meant I was high as a kite and pretty pleased about everything! I remember giving the woman next to me, who had undergone shoulder surgery, the full rundown of how I would be back playing in no time. I'm not sure she appreciated it.

I returned to playing cricket at around five to six months. All of my rehab was done with the Redbacks. There was a step-by-step program and process for me to follow before being allowed back to playing cricket including consultation between the surgeon, physio and strength and conditioning team. All was mapped out and well planned. Everyone worked together.

Despite the great rehab and support, I was still nervous about my return. In cricket we wear steel spikes on the bottom of our shoes, and they grip strongly. The grounds then were mostly couch grass which is quite tightly knitted. It's not as common these days, mainly because it's known as a potential cause for knee injuries. Instead, they now use a thinner turf with slightly moist soil, so there is a bit of give in the ground. But back then, with the tightly knitted grass of the Adelaide Oval, I did feel a bit anxious. I was particular about my footwear and didn't like having spikes that were too long or too new.

At no point did I wear a brace. I asked about it early on, and my physio said a brace would be more of a mental aid rather than any structural need. The minute he said that, I thought, 'I don't want it'. I believed I could be strong enough mentally to handle not wearing one.

After my rehab ended, we tried to be as proactive as possible. The thought was that as I had naturally hyperextending knees this would leave me predisposed to potential further ACL injuries. With that knowledge I have always had some knee-specific exercises in my exercise program that perhaps some others don't. That gave me added confidence—the fact I was doing a little more on my legs and for my agility just to make sure I was sharp. I was giving myself every chance.

There was one instance, late in my comeback season, when my knee had a slight instability episode. I went to field a ball and I felt it give just a touch. It made me a bit nervous, but I got over it pretty quickly. That was the only moment I felt any issue in the five years between my first and next ACL injury.

Four years after that initial injury, I was selected in the Australian one-day cricket team. I played 27 games before reinjuring my knee and was left out of just one game to rest and give another player a go. I was proud of the fact I'd been able to nail down a spot in the team, then ranked number one in the world. I was learning a lot from guys like Ricky Ponting, Michael Clarke, Mike Hussey—it really felt like things were going well for me. My four-day cricket was also starting to come along, and I was heading in the right direction to get to where I wanted to be— the Test team.

We were playing New Zealand in the 2009 Champions Trophy final in South Africa, when I reinjured my right knee. I had been battling some quad problems for a few weeks leading into this tournament. I'd reached the point where I was wearing compression sleeves on both quads and having daily physio, and I was really wondering whether I'd be able to get through games. It felt like I had constant knots in my quads, and I was having to find ways to run that wouldn't put too much strain on them.

In the final I was fielding at mid-off, and the ball got hit to cover. Ricky Ponting dived and got a hand to it, which then knocked it to my right. I stepped forward to pick up the ball to throw it across my body at the stumps, and my right knee gave way. I sort of kangaroo bounced over it. I hit the deck and knew straight away what had happened. I felt that tearing sensation again. Not a pop, just a tear. Mitchell Johnson was yelling at me to throw the ball, but I wasn't going anywhere. It was three overs from the end of the innings, when I would have been putting on the pads to bat, but I didn't make it through the fielding innings.

I came off and made it up the Centurion Grandstand stairs (all 5361 of them it felt like!) to the change rooms. I thought maybe I was okay, because within 15 minutes I was doing arse-to-grass squats with no pain. But my knee was lax when the physio did the ligament tests. When it came to the batting innings, the physio strapped my knee as tight as possible as Ricky Ponting wanted me to go in at number eight if needed, to hold up an end. It got to the point where I had my pads on, but I wasn't required. We got the runs and won the tournament without me having to go out and bat, which was probably a good thing. I could have been in a bit of trouble facing some of their fast bowlers with a poorly functioning back leg.

The team physio organised for me to see a surgeon in Johannesburg the next morning. He drew some fluid out of my knee and there was blood in the syringe, so he was fairly confident my ACL had been ruptured. That was a real downer.

I flew home with the team and reconnected with the same surgeon and physio. An MRI scan confirmed my ACL was gone, and so I proceeded to have a full reconstruction using a hamstring graft. The surgeon talked about a patella tendon graft but felt that for me the hamstring was the safer option. LARS grafts were also around at that stage, but that certainly wasn't the way anyone in the room was keen to try. There was also a bit of cartilage damage, but not as bad as the first time. The operation went well, and I got stuck into the rehab phase unhampered.

There were a few more players in my support team this time around. I had an additional layer of support and professionalism with the physio from the Australian team checking in regularly on my progress. We also 'cross-pollinated' and I spent some time with a knee rehab specialist at the Geelong AFL club.

My second rehab was a lot more involved. This allowed me to get my confidence up quickly and to really push my boundaries. I'd been around a while now, so things had changed a lot since my first experience. Sports science research had progressed, and everyone's rehab was improving. I started doing trampoline work, and other things I hadn't done the first time around. As part of my ongoing maintenance and preparation I was now including a lot more plyometric-type training with jumping and landing, hopping, and gymnastics style stuff. It was fantastic. I really enjoyed it.

I returned to playing practice matches at around 10 months. I played my first professional game with the Redbacks at eleven-and-a-half months after the surgery. But it wasn't until around another 12 months after I returned to playing professionally that I started to feel 100 per cent again in my movement patterns on the field.

In December 2015, I was playing for the Melbourne Renegades. I'd had the best first half of the Sheffield Shield season I'd ever had, with nearly 500 runs in five games. I'd just posted my highest first-class score—213 against Tasmania, and then a few weeks later, I injured my other ACL.

We were playing at Junction Oval in Melbourne, and I was at deep square leg. The ball was hit to my left and rolling along the outfield, so I sprinted as hard as I could. I went to hop around the ball to pick it up on my right side so I could throw it in quicker. As I hopped, I landed on my left leg and my top half kept turning while my spikes got stuck in the ground. It was a tightly knitted couch grass, and my spikes just got stuck in there. I kind of kangaroo bounced again over my leg as the knee hyperextended and I felt that tearing sensation again. I went down and wasn't getting up in a hurry. I knew straight away. It was probably the most aggressive mechanism in my three episodes. I wasn't overly confident I was going to come out of it well.

An MRI organised for the next day confirmed my ACL was gone. I flew back to South Australia and saw my original surgeon again. He was away on holidays but did me a massive favour by coming back early to perform my surgery. I knew the importance of not letting my muscles waste away by getting on the operating table quickly, especially after the delay I experienced years back after being misdiagnosed in Bangladesh. My muscles just wasted away in that time, and I pretty much lost everything. Still to this day, my right leg struggles to maintain its quad size. The fact my surgeon came back from his holiday and operated within a few days of the injury meant that I didn't lose a lot of muscle mass in my left leg. A hamstring graft was used again, and there was a bit of cartilage damage, but not as bad as I'd had in the right.

My rehab was again done in South Australia and was pretty similar to my previous one. I had my original physio, and a new strength and conditioning coach who had a strong AFL background with ACL-rehab experience. I had an experienced team of sports science professionals around me, along with a gymnastics coach. I couldn't have asked for better support.

This time it took me just under 11 months to get back to playing professionally. I had more confidence going from one step to the next. I also didn't have as much time to be ready for the first game of the season as I'd had previously. But I returned in good form and was subsequently selected to make my Test debut against South Africa in Hobart in November 2016. After a poor performance however, I was dropped. It was my only Test match.

My knees don't limit me at all now with my cricket. They don't hyperextend as much as they did before the surgeries—I'd say they are straight now—but when stretching, my heel doesn't get to my butt on either side. It's not a problem, but I notice my quads are really tight much of the time. I was able to get most of my speed back after each of the three operations, but my full flexion range just isn't quite there. Even now, physically I feel as though I have a few years left in me, if I decide to keep playing.

REFLECTIONS

Looking back, each of my ACL experiences was unique and taught me different things. Being only 18 with my first ACL injury, it didn't feel like the end of the world. People around me were saying cricket had a low risk of re-injury, it being less aggressive on your body compared to sports such as football—especially for a batter like me. I was in a reasonable head space and had a really good support network around me. I was confident I would be back playing at some stage the next season. As it turned out, with only a partial tear, I was back a lot sooner which was great.

My second ACL injury—my first full rupture—was more of an emotional roller coaster. Playing in the final of the Champions Trophy was a real career highlight. But getting injured on the way to winning it—that was just about as bittersweet as you'll ever get.

I don't think I fully understood what I was missing out on over the next 12 months of my career. I didn't grasp how difficult it was going to be to get back to where I was. Having nailed down a spot in the Australian team, which at that time was the number one ranked one-day side in the world—it was really disappointing to have to step away. I came to realise the challenges you can face when you give up a spot in a side and someone else comes in and makes a real go of it.

My third ACL injury was probably the toughest. Being 29, I was already nudging a little closer to the end of my career than I would have liked. I'd also just had the best first half of a Sheffield Shield season of my career and felt like I was close to getting back to playing for Australia again. To do my other knee—that hit me harder than the previous two injuries, no doubt about it. I remember just breaking down on the phone to my girlfriend Rhiannon (now wife) and family. It was the first time I'd really gotten emotional about an injury.

Despite the setbacks, going through all three of the rehabs left me in a pretty good place and taught me a lot about my body. Not just my knees, but what my body is able to cope with and its warning signs in general. I can better determine the right type of 'sore' from the dangerous type of 'sore'. The whole process gave me a real sense to notice imbalances and weaknesses in my legs, and a good understanding of how to stay on top of those kinds of issues. I realised that even when doing rehab on just one knee, it's important to get both legs to the point where they're equal. If one leg is struggling, then the other is under a lot more pressure which could lead to the good leg being injured.

Going through the tough times with my knees also taught me how to better look after my body in general. I have also kept my fitness at a level that has allowed me to play for as long as I have. I am now in a position where I feel my body could allow me to compete at an elite level for another few years. That's a much longer career than I expected when I first started out.

Injuries are enormously humbling experiences. They do hit you pretty hard. Mine have definitely helped with my empathy and taking notice and more care of fellow teammates. I think that's allowed me to become a good team person and teammate—someone people can talk to. I understand what they're going through and have kept an eye out for them more than if I hadn't gone through those injuries myself. Ultimately, I think my injuries have made me a better person.

I realise how fortunate I've been to be in a high-performance environment with access to an amazing support team. I didn't expect to progress as quickly as I did, particularly in the early stages after the first full reconstruction. The specialist I saw at Geelong Football club was really pushing my knee to a degree I didn't think it was going to be able to stand up to. The hopping and agility work they had me doing really opened my eyes to what my knee and ligament was capable of handling. It was enormously challenging initially, but my confidence went through the roof after the handful of days I spent there. It also excited me because it felt like, 'Wow, if I can do this now, where am I going to be at the end of the rehab?!' The confidence I gained from that short training workshop gave me an enormous boost and the appetite to keep pushing myself to another level throughout the rehab and beyond. To this day I've continued to do a bit of gymnastics-style training whenever I get the chance.

I've also been lucky to have great support from my family and friends throughout. I have a lot of close mates within cricket, but I also had people outside the cricket bubble who I have always found to be a real leveller for me. My wife was an enormous support during the third rehab. She jokes that it was the best thing that ever happened to her—the fact I was able to spend 11 months with her! Between her and my parents, I was waited on hand and foot for the first few weeks after the operations.

For most sports, finding someone to talk to who's been through an ACL reco is relatively easy. But it is enormously rare within cricket. When I first did mine, there had only been one other Australian cricket ACL injury that I knew of, and he is now a coach. For that reason, I reached out to fellow Australian cricketer Usman Khawaja the minute he hurt his. I thought I'd get in touch with him, as there were no other cricketers who have really been through it.

Of all the things I learnt during my ACL journeys, resilience definitely stands out on top. From the first injury onwards, I found little value in complaining or whinging about any type of training. I started to view any sort of physical activity as an investment in my fitness and my body wellness. Any frustrations about having to do an extra fitness session or anything like that didn't bother me. I always saw the positive side. I think people in general would describe me as a very optimistic person, but through my experiences I feel I became even more so.

My advice to others would be to speak to as many people who have been through an ACL rehab as possible. You've got to do as much research as you can yourself, and then work together with a physio with ACL-rehab experience to come up with a program that works for you. I didn't use any magical machines to do my exercises, I was using swiss balls, medicine balls—things that anyone can buy.

A lot of it comes down to internal drive. If you can get into the frame of mind that it *doesn't* mean you're not going to be able to play sport again, you will learn so much. Nothing ever changes with regards to hard work—you put in the effort and you get the rewards. Just commit to looking after your body, and it's amazing how much it will repay you in the long run.

FREESTYLE SKIING

RUSS HENSHAW

Russ Henshaw is a professional freestyle skier who sustained three ACL ruptures during his career—two to his left knee, and one to his right. His choice of management for each injury was unusual—he used his Dad's hamstring tendon for the first graft, and a non-surgical approach for the two subsequent ruptures allowing him to continue skiing at an elite level. He competed at the 2014 Sochi Winter Olympics without either of his ACLs! He then chose to reconstruct both knees simultaneously using cadaver grafts, and skied successfully through another Olympic cycle.

I started skiing when I was three years old. I grew up in south-west Sydney, and we had a unit in Jindabyne that we'd go to in the school holidays. When my parents put me into ski school the instructors quickly suggested they should put me in the race program. Mum and Dad weren't keen initially, but the next year we went back for another family snow holiday, and a different set of instructors said the same thing. So, they enrolled me, and I raced until I was 12. I liked racing, but I liked jumping more—you could tell because I was always taking the long route down to the training course, hitting all the jumps and bumps along the way. Even though I was young, once I decided that racing wasn't for me and swapped over to freestyle skiing, it was just a snowball effect from there.

We moved to Jindabyne permanently around the same time I started freestyle skiing. The move definitely played a huge role in where I ended up in my ski career. I started travelling the world at 14 and became a pro at 15. I wouldn't have had half the opportunities I had presented to me—living in the Aussie snow fields often put me in the right place at the right time. I was lucky to grow up skiing in winters and skateboarding in summers. I never really was one for team sports.

I skied professionally for 12 years competing and filming internationally in slopestyle and big air. Slopestyle is pretty much a skate park running down a hill with lots of features such as jumps, rails, and quarter pipes, and big air is—as the name suggests—a really big jump.

The season before my knee issues began, I was skiing well winning X Games silver, and Dew Tour and World Championship bronze. Despite ongoing knee troubles over the following years, I managed to return to form, winning Dew Tour gold and World Championship silver, and competing at both the Sochi and PyeongChang Winter Olympics. I retired from skiing in 2018 and moved back to Jindabyne to start the next chapter of my life—carpentry and fatherhood. These days I enjoy skiing at home in Australia for the fun of it.

I've definitely had my fair share of injuries over the years. My left ankle had an avulsion fracture. I've broken my collarbone. Broken my wrists. Broke my hand. I've torn my right ACL twice, and my left ACL once. I also shattered my left kneecap so badly the doctors couldn't count how many pieces it was in.

The first time I blew my ACL was at the end of probably the best northern winter season I'd had. I was 22 at the time. I'd placed second in X Games, third at Dew Tour, and had a bunch of other results. I felt invincible. At the end of the season we were filming a spring park shoot in Alaska. I had done all of the tricks I wanted to do for the film, so decided to try a new trick I'd been practising on the trampoline and give it a whirl on the jump. The trick went ok, but there was a foot of slushy snow on landing the jump which my skis sunk into as my body kept rotating. My binding didn't release because I had the DIN setting (the value for setting the releasability of the ski binding) cranked pretty high. That season I'd pulled a bunch of skis off in the air from pulling a grab too hard, and as a result had some pretty hectic crashes. I didn't want to keep pulling my ski off mid-air, so I'd wound the DIN up a little. It's always a bit of a fine line you dance with when skiing.

I didn't feel a pop. I have never felt that with my ACLs. I was in pain for about 30 seconds, then it went, and I felt fine. I could walk. I could do everything. But by that night, my knee was massive. It was then I realised something wasn't right. I got it checked out in Alaska, and they said it was loose, but they weren't sure about my ACL because the swelling made it harder to do the testing.

It was the end of the season anyway, so I changed my flight and flew home to get it checked out. Once back in Australia, I saw my surgeon and had an MRI that showed the ACL was gone. Luckily for me it was a clean snap, there was no other major damage.

We then decided to go about things in a rather unique way. For all of my surgeries, I've never had any of my hamstrings taken. I guess that started from this first one. My surgeon gave me the option of doing a donor allograft. The donor was my dad. We used his hamstring for my ACL, to potentially speed up my recovery time, and not compromise my hamstring function. We did discuss other graft options, but for me this seemed like the best one at that time. Just the idea of not having two separate injuries to deal with—as in having to rehab the hamstring graft site as well—made it seem like the best option. A conservative approach was never discussed. It was either have the surgery or stop skiing. My career was just starting to take off, so I was pretty keen on not having to stop.

I had surgery at the end of May 2011 and took the Australian season off and rehabbed in Jindabyne. I kept my sanity by judging a couple of events, and if there were film shoots happening, I would go up the hill. Although I wasn't skiing, I still managed to stay involved with my friends and the industry.

I had a pretty epic local Jindabyne team as far as my physio and trainer. I was flipping to and from Sydney to see my surgeon, but most of my rehab was done in Jindabyne. There was no formal testing for a return to snow, but I passed everything they set for me, and made sure I could do it all before letting myself return to snow. I didn't want to rush it or have in the back of my head that I couldn't do something.

I was back on snow in just under six months and competing at around seven months. I had to hit it pretty hard, and pretty quickly because it was the start of the qualifying year for the Sochi Winter Olympics. I flew to Austria and stayed with my team manager and skied groomers for two to three weeks to start with. I forced myself to go skiing where there was no terrain park (the area at a ski field with jumps and rails) so I wouldn't be tempted. There were just groomers in Austria, so it was perfect. From there I flew to Colorado and had a week or two until the Dew Tour which would be my first competition back. I started skiing in the baby park, but it all progressed pretty quickly from there. I placed third at Dew Tour, and my knee survived. I was happy.

At that point I felt 100 per cent confident in my knee. But I wasn't 100 per cent confident in my tricks because I hadn't been skiing, trampolining, or jumping for such a long time. I felt rusty and disjointed. My speed management for jumping was off—I found myself overshooting jumps and coming up short. Before the injury I had no issues, I could look at a jump and just know where to drop from. That skill took me a while to get back. I'm not sure why.

I wasn't wearing a brace as I found it really uncomfortable. My surgeon said my knee was strong, and that the brace would just be there as a helper, but it wouldn't make my knee bulletproof. He felt it was my choice to wear one or not. I didn't really want to be the bionic man, so I didn't wear one when I returned to snow.

After Dew Tour we went to Whistler and trained for two weeks. We then headed back to Colorado for another few weeks of training at a Red Bull performance camp. I felt great by then. My speed management was back, and I was doing all of my tricks again. I didn't want to be limited by not ever doing the trick I'd hurt myself on, so the camp gave me the opportunity to relearn that trick before X Games.

During training at X Games, I pretty much had my run dialled. During the last training session, I went to do that same trick again, but went a little too big off the jump. I landed backseat (leaning backwards) with a twist, and felt my knee go again. I knew it straight away. When I stood up, the knee was really sore. That was the end of my X Games campaign.

I flew straight home and saw another surgeon who had been recommended to me this time. He got me to do a bunch of tests. The knee didn't feel unstable. It felt fine. The only times I would really notice it was if I put my foot up on a stool while sitting and let my knee hang; or if I was standing and not really concentrating and went to lock my leg out. It would feel like it wanted to keep going. But I could hop, jump, squat. I could do all of it.

We decided to give the non-surgical approach a go. Initially the conversation was: 'When can we book you in for surgery?' But I explained where I was in my career and the upcoming Olympics and emphasised that my knee didn't feel unstable and I felt fine. There was next-to-no swelling too this time which was bizarre. I also told the surgeon about P. K. Hunder, one of my skiing mates from Norway who had torn his ACL and was successfully skiing and doing the Olympic qualifying without an ACL. We chatted about it and he said, 'If you feel confident, there's no reason you can't do it. You just need to wear a brace'. He wasn't a big advocate for a brace either, but all considering, I was happy to wear one this time round.

I stayed in Sydney for a month or so and my sponsor Red Bull hooked me up with one of Sydney's top conditioning coaches who worked with one of the football teams. He took me on for two one-on-on sessions a day. I then went back to Jindabyne for a few more weeks, and trained with my local trainer and physio, before returning to Mammoth Mountain in the USA for some springtime skiing to prepare for the World Cup event in New Zealand later that southern winter. It was our first Olympic qualifying event.

It was easier returning to snow this time round. When I first got back on skis, I had a little doubt in my mind, but after a week of skiing my knee felt fine. I think one of the main reasons it was easier was because I didn't have the length of time off the snow that I'd needed after surgery. I didn't feel like I'd lost that much that I'd been working on. My tricks didn't feel rusty. I didn't lose my speed management. I just had a brace on this time when skiing, but not when I was in the gym or doing any other training.

By the time I got to New Zealand I was confident in my knee. I only really noticed it if I went too big off a jump. I could feel my joint do a little shift on landing. But it wouldn't hurt. I could just feel it, and it felt pretty gross to be honest! I managed to finish third in New Zealand. And with that result, I'd pretty much done enough for Olympic qualifying after that one event.

I spent the rest of the southern winter skiing in Australia before returning to New Zealand for spring camp. After spring camp, I put more emphasis on gym time, rather than flying straight to the northern hemisphere for glacial skiing like I would have done in the past. I stayed in Jindabyne and trained for a bit longer, before leaving for Colorado at the end of November.

I competed in the Dew Tour and a World Cup event and did well getting podiums at both. The next event was X Games, and I was feeling a million bucks. Training went well. Everything was great. There were no issues with my knee. I made the finals, but on my last run I ran into a head wind which made me come up short on the landing of the first jump. My left knee didn't feel that great after crashing, so I went down and saw the Red Bull medicos who said, 'You're all good, there's nothing wrong'. I wasn't convinced so I got an MRI in Aspen, but they couldn't see anything on the imaging either. From there I pretty much had to hightail it to the airport to fly to Russia for the Olympics.

My knee was swollen, but it didn't feel bad. Through the airport I was jumping around trying to prove to my girlfriend Laura (and myself) that it was fine. I must have looked like an idiot. But I was running and jumping around, even hopscotching down the bridge to the plane. It didn't feel bad. It didn't feel like I'd done my ACL.

Then I got to Russia and saw the Australian doctor. He was pretty adamant I'd done it. But considering I had been skiing without my right ACL for the past season and a half, it was hard for him to tell me I couldn't ski without my left. Although he did try.

There was only three weeks between the X Games and the start of the Olympic Slopestyle event—even less if you counted the training days beforehand. Once I started jumping in training, I wasn't worried about instability. But I realised I was going to have to deal with quite a bit of pain in my knee because of the bone bruising. It was still so fresh and was not impressed with the impact from landing a 20-metre jump. I was pretty confident in my knee, but it was just the pain—when I landed an intense sharp pain would shoot up my femur. During training, I didn't land a single run or link any of my tricks in a top-to-bottom run.

I was wearing a borrowed knee brace that didn't fit well during the training sessions. But I had to make do until a new one arrived from Australia, one that was the same as the one I wear on my other knee. Luckily it arrived two days before my event. My physio was also heavily taping my knee before each day on the snow, and I was spending some serious time every evening icing my knee with the Game Ready.

Despite all of this the Olympics went better for me than I expected. As you can imagine, I had a lot of stuff going around in my head with different people's opinions as to whether I could do it or not. But my idea was that I'd made it this far, I wasn't about to not give it a crack. I had to. So, I did just that. And with a bit of a miracle I got an all right score and managed to make it through to the finals.

In the finals I decided to step it up a notch, but it didn't go my way. My first run got an okay score, but not what I was looking for. My second run was going well, so on the last jump I went for a triple cork (an off-axis triple flip) and I slightly under-rotated and slid out on the landing. That was the end of my first Olympic journey—I ended up eighth.

Although I was pretty chuffed with the result, there were definitely mixed emotions. Looking through one lens, I was proud of my efforts considering all I had been through to get there. To make the finals was awesome, but it was also gut-wrenching to have put in so much time, effort and work, and then have my 'good' knee go three weeks before the biggest event of my career. It was really bittersweet.

After the Olympics I came home and saw my surgeon again. We chose to reconstruct both my ACLs at the same time using cadaver grafts. He used Achilles tendons, explaining they were meant to be two- to three-times stronger than hamstring grafts because of their thickness. The rehab was a little different, as using the cadaver grafts was deemed similar to using a LARS graft, so it was an accelerated rehab program. It was basically three months instead of six. I had the surgery in March, did three months of rehab, and was back skiing by June for the southern season.

After that I didn't have any issues for the next four years. My knees felt great, until I had another crash in competition just before the PyeongChang 2018 Olympics. I caught my edge on a jump take-off and landed on my back, crunching my left knee which was twisted and tucked underneath me. My ACL didn't go, instead I tore a bunch of cartilage. I still made it to the Olympics but wasn't able to perform as well as I would have liked.

After that injury, it wasn't that I thought I couldn't come back—I knew I had it in me because I'd done it so many times. But I had reached the stage that I was sick of being hurt. I was 28, which is pretty good for a free skier. I could well have gone on skiing without competing, and pursue a career in filming, but that was also getting tiresome for me. The other deciding factor that led to me retiring was that I didn't want to hurt my knees anymore and not be able to teach my kids how to ski or for me to run around on a soccer oval. I was starting to look at the big picture, not just to the next season. I was ready and happy to start the next stage of my life.

The thing that plays on me now with my knees isn't ACL-related. It's my kneecap that I shattered when I was 15, and the bone-on-bone that resulted from my last injury. They just so happen to be on the same knee. If I ski now and spend the day jumping, I'm sore at the end of the day and into the next. But I've found with time that's getting better slowly, and I'm not planning on stopping jumping anytime soon.

REFLECTIONS

I wouldn't say there was anything I could have done better. I believe I did everything in my control well enough given the knowledge I had at the time. Accidents happen in my sport. There are very few free skiers and snowboarders who make it out unscathed. Maybe before my first ACL I should have been warming up a bit more, but saying that, I'd been skiing at a high level for eight years before tearing my ACL and I had never had any issues.

When I have hurt myself a lot over the years, it's often been when I've been too keen. There are just little things you need to focus on, and you need to watch what's happening around you. I wasn't very good at doing that in the beginning. I was fortunate when my ACL injuries started happening, I had already built a bit of a name for myself in the sport, so if they were running an event and it was dumping snow or windy, I would take a stand and say, 'I'm not doing it'. It doesn't matter what's on the line, your safety is more important than a couple of World Cup points.

My surgeries were quite different from what other people did at the time. It's not like you have surgery and you're fixed. You have surgery and then you've got to fix yourself. You've got to put in the work. Go to the gym. Do the rehab. I didn't really realise how in-depth that was before my first ACL injury. But I definitely had a grasp of it when it came time for my second and third rehabs. It was probably the bit I was dreading the most! It's not that I didn't like working out, I just knew how much of a grind it is, and how much you've got to put in.

I had a close friendship with someone who was skiing well without their ACL, but I still would have asked my surgeon whether I could manage without my ACL. It was so helpful to have a fellow athlete and friend in the same situation that I could bounce questions off, compare experiences, and see how he was dealing with it all. Seeing what my friend was able to do without his ACL definitely added to my confidence.

I had a great relationship with my physio. I'd worked with her from when I was a grommet, and she knew me and my previous injuries. She knew my body. You want to be with someone when you go through an injury like this that you've worked with before and have confidence in. I trusted whatever she would tell me and I would listen. If you go into it and do everything you're told to do, you shouldn't have to look back and think, 'Uh oh, I should have done ...'.

There are times when your ACL is still weak and it's probably not the best idea to do some of the activities you want to do. You might think you're aware of your body, and your body feels good, you feel good, but your physio says, 'You can't do that yet'. That was one of the lessons I learned in rehab that transferred to skiing after—pulling back every now and then is not always a bad thing. If you're feeling weak or fatigued, there's not much point in doing another set, or if you're feeling tired when you first get back on snow—or whatever your sport is—then maybe pull it back a bit. I really learned to listen to my body. A lot more than I used to.

I had a formal warmup program I would do before I went out on the hill. There was also another maintenance program I would do in the gym afterwards. Before I injured my ACL, I did have a warmup, but not to the same level. I wasn't warming up for as long as I should have. I wasn't stretching as much as I should have. The behaviour was there, but the extent wasn't.

I also learned a lot about nutrition and how it plays a part in recovery and performance. I definitely didn't have the strictest diet when I started out. I was a free ski athlete, which back then, meant I was a relatively unconventional athlete. But my injuries taught me about fuelling my system and making sure I didn't compromise that side of things. If you don't fuel right, you won't get what you need out of the hard work you're putting in.

The time constraint I had was never ideal before the Olympics. There's never a good time to hurt yourself, but especially not right before the Olympics. But you can't sit there and dwell on it—if you do, you're not going to achieve anything. I just tried to take the necessary steps to try to get back on the snow and make things happen. That was my approach.

There's always more to consider than just the physical side of an injury. The mental game for me was huge, particularly at the Sochi Olympics. My main support team had always been outside the Australian winter system, but once in Russia I was under the care of the Australian Team. On arrival, I had my knee checked by the team doctor. He was just doing his job, but he didn't know me at all as a person and hadn't been involved in my leadup, aside from quick pre-season testing. He delivered the news to me about my ACL in a really poor way. Any hope I had felt like it was stripped from underneath me. He pretty much said, 'There's no way your leg is going to cope with what you're wanting to put it through'. That was frustrating to hear, to say the least, especially considering I'd just done 18 months of exactly that without my other ACL! Although I hadn't been able to test my knee on snow yet, to me it felt the same as my other knee; it didn't feel unstable. I just wanted to have a go. I wanted to try. My thoughts were that it already needed fixing, and if anything else happened I'd deal with the consequences. But the decision should be mine.

That meeting definitely put me in a pretty poor headspace. It then just became another thing I had to deal with mentally, alongside performing at my best at the biggest sporting event in the world, on the biggest course anyone had ever seen—with no ACLs.

I had been lucky to have my wife Laura travel the ski circuit with me. She was my rock through everything, definitely so in Sochi. She kept me in a positive frame of mind. Pretty much everything she could do behind the scenes she was doing—from the big things to the little things, making me smile, making me not stress, telling me to go with my gut rather than what everyone else was saying. I've never seen a sports psych. It's always just been Laura and my family and friends.

Aside from having a brace on my legs, skiing without my ACLs didn't really feel that much different to having them. I felt I could perform fully and I never had instability issues or collapsing. When I was skiing for the 18 months without my right ACL, if I had a big day on snow, I would end up with a little bit of swelling in my knee. I just had to be more focussed on recovery. I was always on the spin bike and icing up.

I wasn't worried about causing future injuries to my knees. I felt that if I had a big crash, the same damage was probably going to happen whether I had an ACL or not. I was already down that path where my knees would need fixing one day. The way I looked at it was, if I hurt myself again, I would have to have some sort of surgery anyway.

I chose to reconstruct my knees because of the pain from the bone bruising and cartilage in my left knee. I just wanted them to be a bit more secure, I guess. P. K. Hunder however, is still skiing without either ACL after eight years!

If you decide to go down the conservative path, it's not just, 'I don't have an ACL now, but I'll go about my life how I was beforehand'. You've got to change things. You've got to dedicate time in the gym. You've got to dedicate time to looking after yourself, but it has to be dealt with case by case. If I blew my knee today, with where I'm at in life being retired from professional skiing, I'd probably fix it because I don't have the time anymore to spend that amount of time in the gym. I could definitely survive without one, but I'd need to keep working hard in the gym. And that isn't always possible later in life after sport.

If I could give any advice to my former self, aside from 'don't crash!', it would be to just keep having fun. I wouldn't change anything because I wouldn't be who I am today without my experiences. Even though I've had the injuries and had to deal with the pain and the rehab, I've learned a lot about myself and my body, and about what I can and can't do. I know the importance of hard work, resilience, and sticking with what you've started. Those lessons stay with you throughout life. I definitely wouldn't change any of it.

My advice to anyone who has done their ACL, is it's not the end of the world. There's a big perception about it being a game-ending injury, but you know what, it's just a long injury. Stay positive. It's a big learning curve. Take in all the information you can. If this book existed when I was going through it all, it would have been the first thing I would have bought, as there's a lot of information out there, but it's not all good information.

Listen to the doctors and physios and do everything they say to a tee. Try and have fun through the process, because if it's a drag, then it's going to feel like it's taking a lot longer to get back to where you were.

SAILING

ELIZA SOLLY

Eliza Solly is an Australian sailor who has sustained two ACL ruptures—one to each knee. Her first injury occurred while sailing as she aimed for Olympic qualification, and her second playing Australian Football recreationally. Hamstring grafts were used in each of her reconstructions, with the same surgeon and physiotherapist, but with two different rehabilitation scenarios—one as a fully funded elite athlete, and the other as a self-funded recreational athlete.

I joined the Australian Sailing Team in 2013 after finishing school and went straight into campaigning for the Rio 2016 Olympics, sailing the women's 49erFX. It's one of the fastest Olympic boats and requires two people to sail it. My job as crew was to be at the front changing and trimming the sails, while my partner—the skipper—was at the helm steering. We came into the Olympic cycle with a lot of support around us, and achieved top five and top 10 positions at World Cup events, but it wasn't enough; unfortunately, we weren't selected. I continued sailing the 49erFX for the next 18 months, but soon realised I needed a break from the hectic full-time schedule of Olympic sailing. I moved into sailing Etchells—another international class of boat, but not an Olympic discipline—and competed in the 2018 World Championships in Brisbane. I still compete in Etchells sailing, along with other keel boat racing and sailed in the 2021 Rolex Sydney-Hobart Yacht Race.

I was always athletic, taking part in all school sports and lots of netball and athletics. I was very competitive in everything. But my life definitely evolved around boats and the water. My parents were sailors, as were my grandparents, and we had our first family trailer sailor boat when I was around 18 months old. We would spend every holiday down on the Gippsland Lakes. I learned to sail on Port Phillip Bay at Black Rock Yacht Club in lots of different types of boats, before moving onto the 49erFX.

I was never really injury prone as a child. The biggest problems I had were a lot of growing strains and niggles in my knees and heels when I was younger doing Little Athletics. I hadn't hurt myself significantly before my knee.

I injured my right ACL in 2015. It was in the lead-up to a World Cup event in Weymouth in England. We were out on the water training. It was a simple tack—where the boat changes direction through the wind and the crew and skipper move to the other side of the boat. It was a movement I'd done fifty thousand times. I ducked underneath the sail, and as I came out to the other side of the boat and pivoted on my foot, my foot stayed planted as I turned. I felt excruciating pain in my right knee. I screamed and sank down. The pain quickly disappeared and so I laughed it off.

I didn't really know what had happened, I just knew I'd done something to my knee. I didn't feel an obvious pop, maybe more of a rip or a crack. But I was wearing a really thick wetsuit at the time, so that might have dampened what I could feel or hear in my knee.

Our coach came over in the coach boat, and we were all a bit confused as to what had happened. It wasn't like I had slipped, or that it obviously looked as though I'd injured myself. Everything was controlled, and it was a manoeuvre we'd done thousands of times before—nothing out of the ordinary. It was just me moving through the boat as I normally would, but then collapsing; and screaming. Since we weren't sure as to what exactly was going on in my knee, we decided to call it a day. I sat on the bottom of the boat protecting my leg as we sailed in.

When we got into shore I changed out of my wetsuit and there was no obvious swelling. I was a little hesitant to walk on it, but it didn't hurt at all. Our team physio at that event initially couldn't pinpoint exactly what was wrong. He did the Lachman's test, but found both of my knees hard to assess and struggled to get a conclusive feel, even on my good leg. He didn't rule anything out, and did mention my ACL, but as my knee hardly had any swelling at this stage (around two hours after the injury) he was uncertain. He suggested I go home, apply ice, and come back for further assessment in the morning.

I got out of bed, but as soon as I stood up my leg collapsed. That's when I started to think something was really wrong. There was a little bit of swelling, but still not much of a difference from my good side.

Contact had been made with the head Australian sailing physio overnight, and I was set to see a specialist sports doctor in London, two hours on the train from Weymouth. The specialist did all of the knee tests and was pretty sure I'd done my ACL. He organised an MRI, and then sat me down with the results. He started by showing me the MCL on the same leg, which was all the same whitish colour, and then, 'This is your ACL …' which showed black everywhere and lots of disjointed lines. 'It's a full rupture,' he said. I burst into tears.

I Skyped mum and dad on the train on the way back to Weymouth. Dad couldn't believe it. 'You can't do your ACL sailing!' he said. I sent him the MRI report which he then forwarded to his surgeon to check! Dad had done his ACL in the past.

The London specialist suggested I head back to Australia, which

I did at the end of the week. I was lucky to be in great hands. Our head physio had organised everything for when I landed back in Melbourne—from a wheelchair for getting around airports, crutches on the plane, to appointments soon after I landed with my surgeon and the physio who would be taking care of my rehab in Melbourne. (Our head physio was based in Sydney).

I was booked for surgery one week after I arrived home (two weeks after the injury). This allowed me to do some prehab to reduce the swelling and increase the movement of my knee. We discussed different graft types—patella, LARS, and cadaver—and my surgeon explained the background of each one, but he kept coming back to the fact he thought using my own hamstring graft was the best option for this situation. So that's what we did.

My surgery was in June 2015, and the Olympics were in August 2016. We hadn't been selected for the Olympics yet, and the selection regattas were taking place between November 2015 and February 2016. Time was tight, but everyone thought it was still possible.

The majority of my rehab was done in Melbourne, my hometown. The initial stages were mostly guided by my physio. I followed his ACL protocol and ticked off all of the tests in each phase before moving on to the next. As things progressed there was also a lot of assistance from our Victorian Institute of Sport (VIS) strength and conditioning coach. My program changed to include more proprioception, jumping and hamstring work than what I had done before I was injured. He also tried to replicate what I had to do in the boat and made me a land-based simulator—a wooden frame the same shape as our boat with replica wires and sails—for me to practise the movement of going from one side of the boat to the other. I was very lucky to have such great resources available to me.

Sailing however, is something you never fully replicate, and I just had to be strong in general to be ready to return to the water. All I was focussed on for the first four or five months was getting my knee better so I could be in the best shape physically. By the time I returned to the water I was probably the fittest I'd ever been.

The final decision as to when I was allowed to return to the water came from our head sailing physio in Sydney. Even though I had ticked off all the boxes on paper, when the assigned date for my return to sailing came, I was so nervous. Deep down I just didn't feel right. Our physio suggested I wasn't ready and to aim for next week. That delay really flicked a mental switch inside me and helped me pass over my mental hump and feel ready again to go sailing. I knew that if I was trying to protect my knee or wasn't in the right frame of mind to go sailing again, it just wasn't going to go well. That extra week was a good thing for me.

I returned to sailing at four and a half months post-surgery wearing a custom knee brace. Our physio made sure we carefully controlled the sessions. I had to write down the intensity and length of each session, and we monitored it that way. We started with 40 minutes for the first session with not much manoeuvring or drills and increased the length and intensity from there.

My first competition was the Nationals at six months post-op. I was still wearing my brace. As I had been doing such a normal movement when I injured myself, the brace helped me to get over the mental hurdle of 'this could happen anytime'. Apart from that I felt fine.

The World Championships were in February in the USA. I was in a really good physical place. I had worked on myself 150 per cent; but the results didn't come. We had a final Olympic selection opportunity a few months later in France, but we didn't get the result there either. And so that was the end of our Olympic campaign.

Disappointed, I returned home and resumed my training at the VIS. I wasn't really sailing. I needed a break. My boyfriend suggested having something to look forward to, so I set my sights on completing a marathon in November. It felt good to put my focus into running. From then on, my knee was fine. It felt the same as my other knee and I was able to finish my first marathon.

A friend asked me to sail with her, and we sailed together on the FX for the summer of 2016/17. She suggested we campaign for the Tokyo

Olympics and so we sailed together for the next 12 months, but it just didn't work out. We had different ways of going about the campaign, and I was just burnt out. After the summer of 2017/18 I faced probably the hardest moment of my sailing career: I decided to stop sailing.

At that point all I wanted was a normal life. I had gone straight from finishing year 12 to sailing full-time and campaigning for Olympic selection. I just wanted to be a normal 20-year-old with a part-time job, and to finish my uni degree. So that's what I did. I plodded along in a semi-normal life. But then, of course, I started to miss competitive sport.

I started playing social Australian rules football in 2018 with my old high school which had started a team. I didn't have any brothers growing up, so I didn't really know football, but I loved it as soon as I started. I loved the team environment.

I knew football was a potentially risky sport for my knees. I was aware of the FIFA 11 program—an injury-prevention program focussing on the warm-up—and I knew I needed to be doing those exercises to look after my knees, but I just didn't want to do it. I was so burnt out and sick of the elite-athlete life in which everyone is constantly looking at you train and picking on everything you do. I just didn't want to do anymore rehab-style training exercises. I came to playing footy to enjoy sport, and to exercise for the joy of it while still being in a competitive environment.

With that approach I was having a great time. We even made it to the Grand Final! That's when I did my left ACL. It was the second quarter and I was chasing the ball next to my opponent, and I just collapsed. There was no impact or change of direction, I just pushed off my left leg as I was running. I grabbed my knee to my chest and hobbled over to the bench with the help of the trainers. I cautiously tried to jog on the sidelines, and it seemed ok. I felt pain in the back of my leg, but I was being optimistic, telling myself I was fine.

At half-time our trainer was able to check it more thoroughly. She thought it felt a bit lax, but I still didn't think it felt too bad. She asked me to try hopping. I did three hops in a straight line, and it was fine. Then she asked me to hop diagonally. I managed two hops diagonally before my leg collapsed and it sounded like I'd snapped a chicken bone in half. I remember the sound vividly. It was so gross. I collapsed on the floor and knew then what had happened. Our team went on to win the Grand Final. It was great to have been a part of that, in some capacity.

I went to a GP to get an MRI referral. I remember the GP commenting on how pragmatic I was about the whole thing. But I knew exactly what had happened, and I knew what was ahead of me, but I wasn't under the elite sport support bubble this time though. I knew I had to get through this one on my own.

I had the MRI done within a few days and called my surgeon as soon as I had the results. I was told he had a waiting list of nine months. Luckily as I was a past patient, they were able to fit me in after a few weeks because of a cancellation. My surgeon was lovely, but also straight down the line, so the conversation around this ACL injury was done pretty quickly. We decided on a hamstring graft again. My previous physio also had a massive waiting list, but I was again able to get an appointment after a few weeks. I was fortunate to still have relationships with my surgeon and physio, otherwise I can imagine things might have taken a little longer to swing into action.

My surgeon had no doubt that I required another surgery. My physio explained how research surrounding conservative and surgical outcomes had progressed since I'd had my first surgery. Although he outlined that non-surgical management was an option, he wasn't 100 per cent happy with that route for me because I was only 23 and I still wanted to ski and do change-of-direction sport.

The first time I had the Olympics as a goal, and a tight timeframe which really made the decision for me; this time I didn't have any time constraints. Since I'd had such a positive rehab experience with my first ACL, I wasn't hesitant to have another surgery even though I knew what was ahead of me. I knew my right knee felt completely normal now, and I was sure the same thing would happen with my left. I didn't want my knee to inhibit me in the future.

The biggest thing we had to work around was to be ready for the Etchells World Championships. They were in October 2018, and I had injured myself in August. My surgeon wasn't happy to do surgery and for me to then participate in a sailing regatta so soon. He felt if I rehabbed and wore a brace, he would be happy to do the surgery *after* the regatta. I had another custom brace made. The maker remembered me, and gave me a discount, but I still had to pay a hefty fee for the brace compared with the first one which had been covered by the Australian team.

I managed to sail in the Worlds with no ACL, and my knee felt fine during the regatta. I did all of my strength exercises in the lead-up, and wore the brace while on the water. I just had to be cautious with my movements. Compared to the physically demanding speed and strength of the 49erFX, Etchells racing suited my knee—it is more about tactics and decision-making. I still had to change sides of the boat with each tack, and pivot and twist as I jumped across under the boom, but it was a more controlled movement. The boat was also much narrower, so I felt safer because I had something to hold onto if I needed to. We came 21st in a fleet of around 100 boats. It was a good result for us. We had a lot of fun, so we were happy.

I had my surgery in November 2018, right before uni break. Compared to my first knee rehab, I wasn't putting as much priority on looking after my leg. I was just going about my daily life and focussing on all the things I missed out on when I was sailing full-time. I went back to working in retail less than a month after the surgery. There was a stool there, so I could sit down if I needed, but I was mostly on my feet. By the end of the day my knee would be so swollen.

I was fortunate to have private health insurance for my second surgery. I'm not sure of the total out-of-pocket costs, but I know for my right knee it was over $10,000 as I had to keep track of it for an insurance claim. My physio and I had a discussion at the start of my second rehab. He knew

I was paying privately and had a life to live now which wasn't 100 per cent focussed on my knee and rehab. During the first rehab I would see him every one or two weeks, but during the second rehab I saw him every month initially and then just every six to eight weeks to keep me accountable. We still ticked off the stages of the ACL rehab protocol, but we tested them less formally than the first time. It was all a bit more relaxed and flexible as he was happy to adapt the end stage rehab to whatever lifestyle I wanted.

After the second surgery, I felt it was too risky to return to footy. I liked footy, but I wasn't 100 per cent invested in it. I thought about playing social netball, and my physio didn't say no, but instead asked if that was really what I wanted, given the risk. We talked a lot about risk versus reward, and he let me weigh it up and decide for myself. I was also into cycling. When it came to doing my single-leg squat test, I scored really well and he said, 'Eliza, that's nearly track cyclist level'. He was gently leaning me towards other sports.

I realised at around 12 months post-surgery that my knee still wasn't feeling 100 per cent. My right knee took under six months to get back to normal, but with my left it was turning out to be more like double that time. I'd say that was reflective of the effort I was putting into my rehab. For my right knee, my entire life revolved around rehab, and it paid off. But when it came to my left, I was doing the exercises three times a week. I was *just* ticking the box. I knew then that I had to put more focus into it as I didn't want to have a gummy knee for the rest of my life.

Around the same time, it also started to sink in more seriously that I have a predisposition to injuring my knees. That I was more likely to injure my ACLs again. That thinking motivated me to do more rehab and strength work, even just little things each week. I still do them—they're part of my weekly strength routine. I always add them in at the start, or before running.

These days I do a lot of cycling and running, and I am planning on doing some triathlons. Although I am not currently doing anything overly competitive, I keep reminding myself I'm only young, and have had a lot of things squished into my late teens and early twenties—elite sport, injuries, burnout. I'm now just happy trying to live an active and normal life.

REFLECTIONS

When I was told I'd done my ACL the first time, I burst into tears straight away. I was completely distraught. I immediately thought about sailing, and how I was letting my skipper down as well. I knew that an ACL was a pretty extensive injury, as my dad had ruptured his in 2005, so I had some idea of what I was in for. I knew it wasn't just a six-week recovery.

I was a very different person back then. I was a young girl who followed everyone's guidelines. I was so naïve. I didn't really think for myself, I just followed what everyone was saying: 'You can get through this'. Also, from my support team: 'We're going to get you there'. I didn't really know if what we were trying to do in the time we had was achievable, but when my physio told me of athletes who had returned to Olympics in four months, it was motivating for me. I feel the scenario was a little sugar-coated, but I realised that is what needed to happen when you're campaigning for an Olympics.

The second time my reaction was very different. It was more like: 'Okay, this has happened'. No emotions. Let's just get it done. I think that was because I knew what I was in for. I knew the surgery and rehab was something I just had to get over and done with.

Although the time between the two injuries wasn't large (I was 20 when I injured my right ACL, and 23 my left), I was at very different stages in life. That changed what I learned from each one. My first ACL rehab taught me to become better at listening to my body as every day was different. Some days I'd be able to do my rehab five times over and I'd be fine, and other days I'd just have to sit there with an icepack on and off all day. It also taught me just how resilient my body is, and although it sounds clichéd, that when you put your mind to something you can really get it done. It proved to me that I could achieve anything. It also highlighted my attention to detail and how anal and obsessive I can be when given the chance. Everything from my rehab protocol to nutrition was broken down into very simple tasks right from the beginning, from getting up in the morning, doing a 10-minute set of exercises, to making a smoothie with a whole lot of amino acids in it. They were all really simple things, but as I ticked them off, I could see the results. And at the end of the process, I had managed to achieve something that most people said was impossible. I was back on the water at before five months, rather than the nine months my sceptics had forecast. I knew what I'd done to get myself there, so that was a good little confidence boost.

Having the second ACL injury really forced me to reflect more deeply. It kept on bringing back everything that had happened to do with my right leg which was then all to do with sailing. It made me realise I hadn't had any closure from my Olympic sailing career. So the learnings were different second time around. The left knee was more to do with personal development and me being in charge of myself. The experience really helped me to grow as a person.

The training environments between the two rehabs could not have been more different. The VIS is great because you are training with all kinds of athletes. I was able to speak with and work out with a netballer who had also injured her ACL and had surgery two months before me. It was great to have such a motivated rehab partner, and I could chase her progress along the way. The second time around, I had a friend who was a month or so ahead of me in her ACL rehab, but I was telling her what to do. She wasn't as committed or as understanding of the rehab process, so it was different not having other athletes with an elite background to relate to.

I remember initially thinking that ACL rehab would be more of a timeline thing—at two weeks you can do X, then at four weeks you can progress to Y. I was so frustrated at one of my early physio appointments because he wasn't letting me progress my exercises. But my physio was great. He printed off the protocol and asked me to read the stages. There was nothing about timeframes. He told me not to think about it in terms of time, but rather in stages. I had to tick off each stage before I could progress to the next. He wanted me to understand the process and know what was going on. That was really helpful for me once it was explained that way.

I explained that to my friend the second time around, as I think she kept comparing herself to me. She was always saying things like: 'But you're already doing this'. I would continually tell her that you've got to go through your own stages, and when you can get one stage done you can then move onto the next. I think most people I have spoken to with ACL injuries over the years have found that helpful.

Both of my knee injuries were isolated ACL injuries. I had a grade 2 MCL strain on my first injury, but there was no meniscus or cartilage damage in either, yet my experiences after the two surgeries were quite different. My first knee hardly had any swelling, but for my second knee, my entire lower leg from my ankle to my knee was black for a few weeks afterwards. Right from the word go I just felt like the second one wasn't as smooth. I wasn't fully invested in it, I didn't have all of the resources, and my leg's reaction to the surgery was so much more extreme. My left knee is still a bit short of 100 per cent. It still fatigues a little bit quicker, and my hamstring strength isn't quite there.

My biggest supporters throughout both injuries were definitely my family—my Mum and Dad, and my boyfriend. My physio was also amazing. The first time he was great with the performance side of things—to get back for the Olympics and in helping my confidence. And when I did my second knee, he really helped me put everything into perspective.

Thinking about what didn't go well the first time, it would be that my focus was very much on my individual rehab and performance. The sailing partnership with my skipper was neglected. When you're sailing a double-handed boat you obviously need to have a really good relationship with the person you're sailing with, so you can perform and compete in high-pressure situations. Because I had injured myself, we weren't spending time together. She lived in Sydney, and I lived in Melbourne, which didn't help. I had such an intense rehab to focus on, while she was just left waiting for me. That really affected our team dynamic.

The only thing I would change with my left knee would be to better prioritise my lower leg conditioning and knee preparation coming into playing footy. There's just so many footy injuries for girls. I know I should have done more rehab and prep work (such as the FIFA 11 program) when I was playing footy.

Had I also paid more attention to my family history perhaps I could have been more careful to avoid knee injuries in the first place. I suspect there is a genetic component for me as, on both sides of my family, there is a history of ACL injuries. Dad ruptured his skiing. He didn't even crash, he just hired a different pair of skis from those he normally skied on, and on the first turn it tore. My cousin on my mum's side also did his playing rugby, and his mum (my aunt) also did hers skiing.

I was on the combined pill when I first did my knee. I was on it to be able to manipulate my cycle around the competitive season, as well as for contraception, and for my skin. I can't remember where I was in my cycle when I did my ACLs, and no one ever asked me. When I did my first ACL, our head physio suggested I go off the pill for flying and surgery due to the increased chance of blood clots, but there was never any discussion around my menstrual cycle and the risk of knee injury. I know now that there is some link with increased laxity in your ligaments when you're on your period, but when I was sailing the sport was very male-dominated. There were no female coaches, and I never discussed my menstrual cycle with anyone, not even my female sailing partner. In my experience periods weren't discussed at all in our sport. Looking back now that does seem somewhat ridiculous.

If I could offer any advice to my former self it would be to not be so hard on myself. To better acknowledge and celebrate the small steps along the way. My advice to others would be to know where your finish line is, but to not focus solely on it. You need to focus on each small step, day by day. And of course, try to keep things interesting, as a lot of the rehab can be quite repetitive.

ICE HOCKEY

NATHAN WALKER

Nathan Walker is a professional ice hockey player who has twice undergone surgery for his right knee—an arthroscope for meniscal damage, and four years later an ACL reconstruction using a patella graft. His management and rehabilitation were predominantly USA-based, with a short stage of rehabilitation in Australia during his off-season.

I play professional ice hockey and was the first Australian to be drafted and play in America's National Hockey League (NHL). When I was 13, I moved from Sydney to the Czech Republic where I played in the Czech *Extraliga* League for five and a half years. I then moved to North America where I've been playing since 2013. I am currently contracted with the St Louis Blues. I previously played with the Washington Capitals, where we won the Stanley Cup in 2018. So far, I've played more than 500 professional games in my career, and I'm hoping I have a lot more left in the tank.

Growing up in Sydney I played cricket, rugby league, rugby union, and inline hockey. I started playing ice hockey when I was around five years old. There was a drop-in league at our local rink, and my brother and I decided to give it a go. We loved it. From then on all I wanted to do was play. All day. Everyday.

Ice hockey isn't the easiest game in which to excel at in Australia. It's a lot easier to buy a football and boots from the local sports store than get fitted out with ice hockey equipment. Add to that the difficulty in finding rinks, the end result is small participation numbers and a lower level of competition here compared to Europe and North America. At 13, I was already playing in the under 13s, under 15s, and under 18s, and there just wasn't enough ice time available for me. I decided to chase the dream of becoming a professional hockey player and moved to the Czech Republic.

My Sydney coach had a contact in Czech and was able to set me up for a week-long tryout with the junior team at HC Vitcovice. They decided to give me a go, and I was lucky enough to be taken in by a local ice hockey family whose child also played at the same club. They didn't really speak English, and I didn't speak any Czech, so it was difficult to find out what we were having for dinner! It wouldn't have been easy taking in a 13-year-old who didn't speak the language or really know anything about their country. I will always tip my hat to them for that.

Before my ACL I'd mostly had niggly muscle injuries, nothing too serious. When I was 17, in 2011, I did have a meniscus cleanout in my right knee. It was a bit of a weird one; I woke one day, and my knee didn't feel so good. It only required a quick scope and I was back playing in no time. But ice hockey is a rough game, and in recent years I've had a few more injuries. I've broken my big toe, a bone in my hand, and a bone in my neck. I've also had an osteochondroma in my left knee cut out, which is like a cauliflower growth of extra bone. I also recently suffered a grade 2 PCL tear to my right knee which has been managed without surgery.

The ACL happened in the second year of my professional career. I'd had an awkward collision two weeks earlier, when my right knee twisted.

When I picked myself up and started skating again it just didn't feel right. But I ignored it thinking it would get better over time. Looking back now, I wish I'd stopped to see what was going on with my knee. I was with Hershey [an affiliate of the Washington Capitals] at this point playing in the American Hockey League (AHL), and decided not to seek any medical help, even though it was available. I thought it was just a bruise. Two weeks later I got hit again playing in the East Coast Hockey League (ECHL). It was a shoulder-to-shoulder collision and my right foot was turned out at 45 degrees, and my skate blade stuck in the ice while my knee turned with the rest of my torso. I felt a pop in my knee, but it didn't hurt at all. As I stood up and went to skate, I just had no power or stability. It felt like my lower leg was hanging on by a string. It didn't feel like it was connected to my body. That's when I knew it was pretty bad.

I subbed off and sat on the bench for a few minutes before thinking I'd give skating another go. I went back out, but it was the same thing. I subbed off again, and the doctor evaluated it. He did the pivot shift test and said, 'It feels like you've done your ACL, but let's get an MRI'. Sure enough, a couple of days later the MRI confirmed it was torn.

My surgeon had treated one of our other players with great reviews. I felt confident with him and didn't feel the need to seek a second opinion. He felt my ACL needed to be dealt with surgically, it was just a matter of how we approached it and which graft type to use. He mentioned cadaver grafts can sometimes be rejected by the body, so I didn't want to go down that path. I had a couple of friends who'd torn their hamstring grafts, so that was playing on my mind. It was a bit of a no-brainer in the end for me to go with a patella graft. My surgeon believed it was a stronger graft, and had experience with them, which also made me more at ease. Although he thought the recovery may be a little longer, I was in no rush. I underwent the surgery at the end of January 2015 and didn't need to play again until the beginning of the next season, which began in October 2016.

I also needed to manage my left knee's osteochondroma. My iliotibial band (ITB) was flicking over the bony bump on the outside of my knee.

It wasn't fun, and also needed surgery. That was originally scheduled for the off-season, but as its recovery time was quicker than for the ACL, we decided to bring it forward.

I had the left knee surgery, and a month later, once the swelling in my right knee had gone down, I underwent ACL surgery. Between the surgeries I was still able to train daily on the bike and continue squats and leg press fairly heavy weights. My leg was strong, but my right knee felt really unstable and unpredictable. It collapsed underneath me a few times and I'd never know when it was going to give way—I could definitely tell my ACL wasn't there anymore.

My rehab initially took place with the club's physio in their clinic. Right from the start we set goals around everything—from when I could come off the crutches to hitting certain benchmarks such as riding a bike with no pain, being able to squat 20 kilos, and so on. There were some setbacks where I had to take it slowly for a few days, but it was mostly a pretty straight-forward process.

By around the fifth month I felt pretty comfortable and progressed to running. I had returned to Australia, as I usually do every off-season. My rehab was mostly strength focussed by then, so I continued with my gym programs under my physio's care; I didn't need to touch base with anyone in Australia. I also had a US strength and conditioning coach who would analyse all the stats from each of my workouts.

I returned to America in July, a little earlier than normal, to start skating again. I started on the ice on my own, and then incorporated things into training, and then games. The doctor manually tested the strength of the graft and was happy with it, but we never did formal physical testing. The testing was all incorporated into the rehab stages and we just moved onto the next stage when I was ready. If I wasn't comfortable, I would continue rehabbing for a bit longer. I was cleared to skate with contact around the eight- to nine-month mark.

When I did return to playing, I felt 100 per cent confident in my knee. I didn't wear a brace then, or at all throughout the whole rehab. The doctor didn't want me to, and I didn't feel the need. Having the doctor say the graft felt tight and that everything was 'good to go' helped me overcome that last little mental hurdle. I felt I had a new knee, and it was time to get back to business.

In the early days after returning to playing my knee would swell up sometimes after games. But I could ice it down, and if we had another game the next night, I would sit it out to get ready for the following week. Sometimes it also got a bit stiff or sore around the patella when it was cold outside. Other than that, my knee has been great.

I went on to play in the NHL for the first time in 2018 and scored a goal in my debut match. We also won the Stanley Cup with Washington that same year. All up I think I've played more than 250 games since my ACL, so it's held up really well. To this day, aside from my PCL (which was unpreventable being a contact injury), I haven't really had any problems.

REFLECTIONS

My ACL experience was pretty straight forward. Most things went to plan, and I was happy with my progression throughout the process. But I did still manage to learn a lot along the way.

When I first did my ACL, I didn't know much about knees and how they worked. I didn't know what to expect about the recovery period other than that it would be a lengthy process. Each night I read up on all things to do with knees, and now I know a lot, as well as how to look after my body. I also learned in the first couple of weeks that I can put on a bit of weight—fairly quickly too!

Obviously, I wasn't happy when I was told I'd done my ACL. It took me a couple of days to realise I was going to be out of commission for eight months or so. But it was something I knew I had to deal with. I also knew no one was going to do it for me. I chose to take a pretty positive attitude. I was determined to come back better, stronger, and be more comfortable on the ice than before. I think that really helped me. When I'd have a bad day and my knee was sore and I didn't want to do anything, I just kept telling myself that everything was going to be okay. Once my knee was healthy, I would look back and see that all that rehab I'd done and everything involved in the process had made me a better person, and a better player.

The thing I learned most was to listen to my body and to give it the respect it needs. To know when it's time to have a bit of a break. If my knee does play up now, I take a breath and sit down and just let it do its thing, instead of keeping on going with what I was doing that put it into that position. I know not to push things until they hurt and to expect it to automatically get better.

I definitely look after myself more than I did before my injury. This is possibly also to do with the fact I'm getting older and realise how important it is to take care of my body. You've only got one of everything, and the better you can take care of it the longer you'll be able to survive. Hockey players can keep going until their late 30s to early 40s, so hopefully I can tick on for another 10 years or so.

There are things I continue to do from my rehab—like rolling out and leg extensions. I can't say I do them every day, but I make sure I'm looking after my knee. I stretch now more than I did previously and have weekly yoga as part of my training schedule. I also use foam rollers and release balls at night when watching TV. I don't know if it directly affects my ACL, but I think if I'm a bit more flexible then I'm less susceptible to injuries.

My training now is better than it was before. I'm also a better athlete than before my injury. To train in a certain way and hold it to a certain standard has become a habit embedded in me. If I treated my body before my ACL surgery as I do now, maybe the injury wouldn't have happened. But that's something I'll never know and there's no going back to change it.

No one else in the team was doing ACL rehab when I was going through it, so my rehab was mostly done on my own. The staff who took care of me did an exceptional job. If I had any questions, I could just ask them, so I didn't really feel the need to reach out to others. It was hard to compare my progress against a couple of teammates and friends I knew who had injured their ACL previously. They had their injuries many years before and the rehab processes had changed since then. My wife, family and friends were enough support for me—if I did have a down day, they were there for me at those times.

The ACL rehab was the most challenging of all of the injury rehabs I've been through. There weren't really any unforeseen challenges that came up, it was just challenging in the sense that I had to go through the rehab for so long. At four months it felt pretty good, but there was still another four months until the ligament had healed and 'glued' itself into your body. The long timespan definitely takes its toll. That's where goal setting really helped me stick to the plan.

I had a large piece of paper stuck on a wall and I wrote down my goals as I went along. Whether it was being able to walk by myself at two weeks, or run at four months, meeting each goal and having the satisfaction of ticking it off definitely helped me feel I was accomplishing something.

If I could go back, there's nothing I would do differently. I feel good with my knee now, so I don't see the outcome as being any better than it is.

For anyone who has done their ACL, I would agree that it absolutely sucks and it's a crappy time. But if I had to give advice, it would be to rip into your rehab and give it your all so as to make your knee as strong as you can. Otherwise, it's not going to feel like it did before. It might feel okay for a year or two, but it will slowly deteriorate. Is it really worth risking your whole nine months of rehab by being lazy? Give your body respect and have a positive can-do attitude with your knee, for now and into the future.

PART 3

AFTERWORD

LISTEN AND LEARN

I hope you have enjoyed reading each athlete's ACL journey, and found their varied perspectives on sustaining and surviving the injury both interesting and insightful. I believe their stories will have provided you with a better awareness and understanding of the physical and mental considerations required for optimal ACL injury management.

You may have noticed recurring themes surrounding each athlete's learnings, despite the different managements of their ACL injuries and various hardships faced—these common issues were one of the drivers for me creating this book. I hope you find their advice helpful to your situation, or to others dealing with this injury.

In many ways this book may have raised more questions than it answers. Which graft type is best? How do I know when I'm ready to return to sport? Is surgery even required? If so, then this book can serve its purpose in acting as a conversation starter—opening up the necessary dialogue between patients, surgeons, and therapists to ensure the best decisions are made with regard to patient-specific ACL treatment.

For those of you unlucky enough to have sustained an ACL injury, you will now know what kind of questions you should be asking of your health professionals. And for health professionals reading this, perhaps these stories have heightened your awareness of the discussions you should be having with your clients—if you've not been already!

As highlighted by the athlete's stories, no two ACL injuries or sets of surrounding circumstances are ever the same. Hence, this book has never intended to be a 'how to' manual for ACL rehab.

However, if you were to come away with a 'cheat sheet' of key questions to consider with regard to your ACL injury, it might read something like this:

ACL CHEAT SHEET

Questions to ask if you've injured your ACL:

Although there can be no one-size-fits-all approach for ACL injury management, there are standard questions that must be addressed and rehab guidelines to be followed to achieve the best outcomes.

- Is surgery required? Or could a trial of non-surgical management be an option?
- If surgery is required, what type of graft would be best? What are the pros and cons of each graft option? Is there a preferred graft option for your chosen sport? What graft technique is your surgeon most experienced with?
- What is the expected timeframe to return to your sport? Can you expect to return to your previous level of sport/activity?

Questions to ask your health professionals:

Ideally you will be working closely with a team of medical and rehab specialists throughout your ACL journey—this team will usually include a surgeon, sports physician, physiotherapist, and strength and conditioning (S&C) coach. But it is important to realise not all health professionals are created equal, with varying levels of experience and expertise. Asking the right questions initially can ensure you will surround yourself with a support team that is right for you.

- Do they have experience with ACL rehabilitation, and in particular with your sport?
- How will they get you from where you are to where you need to be? Ask to see a detailed timeline from early to end stage rehab.
- What will your rehab look like? Ask what type of exercises will be done in each phase, and in what kind of environment (home-based, physio clinic-based, gym-based, sport-specific).
- Who will supervise your rehab? Ideally you will have input from both an experienced physiotherapist and S&C coach, who work collaboratively with one another and provide you with supervision and regular reviews throughout the different stages and settings of your rehabilitation.
- What type of testing do you need to complete before your return to running, and then to your sport? Ideally the answer should be based on function ('You'll be ready when you can show me that you can physically complete these tasks'), rather than a time-frame-based answer ('You'll be ready to run at three months, and play sport at nine months').

SETTING YOURSELF UP FOR SUCCESS

It's much easier to achieve your goals if you know what they are from the start! At the beginning of the rehab process be sure to discuss with your health professionals exactly what it is that you aim to return to doing, and when.

A customised approach specific to you and the requirements of your chosen sport, playing position, and/or lifestyle is important, particularly in the final stage of rehab (your return to sport). Only by working together can you ensure you will achieve what you need to.

If access to quality health care providers is geographically difficult—perhaps you live remotely, or you have a particular therapist in mind who specialises in your sport but is based interstate or internationally—access to specialist medical and rehab providers is now easily achieved via online video appointments (Telehealth). This can also be a great way of seeking a second opinion regarding your management or having an ACL specialist oversee your progress from a distance while you complete your supervised rehab with a local therapist.

PREVENT, PERFORM, RECOVER, & REFLECT

Whether it's preventing an ACL injury in the first place, or stopping a recurrence, numerous sport specific neuromuscular training (NMT) programs (listed in the text box opposite) have all been proven to be effective. They also make you perform better—what's not to like! They all consist of simple exercises with minimal requirements of time and equipment—just 15 minutes as part of your warmup, cooldown, or at home. Get to training early if you have to! The vital and common ingredient in their success is consistency of completion. If you don't do them regularly, you won't gain the benefits. It's as simple as that. No excuses. Make them a part of your regular training.

SPORT SPECIFIC NMT PROGRAMS FOR INJURY PREVENTION

International Olympic Committee - 30 different sports

'Get Set – Train Smarter' Injury Prevention App
www.fittoplay.org
On AppStore or Google Play: Get Set - Train Smarter

Soccer/football

Perform + (adults)
www.footballaustralia.com.au/performance/football-australia-perform

11+ (adults)
www.footballvictoria.com.au/sites/ffv/files/2019-05/11plus_workbook_e.pdf

Fundamentals+ (kids)
www.footballaustralia.com.au/performance/football-australia-fundamentals

11+ Kids
www.footballnsw.com.au/wp-content/uploads/2019/04/FIFA-11-Kids.pdf

Netball

The KNEE program
https://knee.netball.com.au

AFL

AFL Prep to Play
https://coach.afl/prep-play-warm
https://resources.afl.com.au/afl/document/2021/09/02/106535ea-a1b8-4d19-b82d-edcfed9a693c/AFLW-Prep-To-Play-Manual.pdf

Rugby Union

Activate program
www.australia.rugby/participate/coach/coaching-resources/world-rugby-activate

But don't forget the importance of other daily habits and factors that play a role in your body's ability to recover from injury and perform well—plentiful sleep, quality nutrition, adequate hydration, levels of stress, your mental health, and your general wellbeing. Even the most perfect rehab program will fall short if you neglect these basic pillars of health.

If you've been unlucky enough to suffer an ACL injury recurrence, ask yourself if there is anything that you could have done differently? Sometimes it may simply boil down to plain bad luck—but maybe you need to take more time, make sure you pass return-to-sport testing, seek a second opinion, train more consistently, address technique issues, or connect with a different support network with more experience in ACL rehabilitation.

LEARN, CONNECT & SHARE

Thanks to the internet, it has never been easier to connect with others about all things ACL-related. Used in the right way, social media can be a great source of information for therapists and ACL injury sufferers alike. Whatever your favourite social media platform, they can all be used as a valuable tool to provide you with relevant information—from communicating the latest ACL research, to providing social support networks of people going through a similar experience, to being a point of contact with ACL specialists who you may wish to connect with.

Following athletes you admire, and who may be sharing their ACL rehabilitation process, can also be helpful and inspiring. Just be sure not to fall into the trap of comparing yourself to others. Their rehab will most likely not mirror yours, as their injury, needs, and scenario will most probably be different—as we have seen from the stories in this book. But to use them as a talking point with your therapist, or to assist with your own motivation towards your rehab—that route I wholeheartedly encourage!

And lastly, sharing or posting comments and reviews about this book on your social media platforms will only help its stories and information fall into more hands. If you know of someone who could benefit from reading this book, please pass it on. In doing so you will not only assist us all in the process of improving our ACL injury experiences, but also help to take Australia off the world leader's board for our high rates of ACL reconstruction and recurrence!

So please, learn from each other.

Look after each other.

And look after your knees.

They will thank you for it!

—Jess Cunningham

ACKNOWLEDGEMENTS

I had thought this book would be a project well suited to the change of pace that came from working on the frontlines of professional sport to being a new mum—one that I could easily complete while my newborn daughter slept. But I soon discovered my daughter was a terrible sleeper, and that writing a book wasn't a quick (or easy) process; nor one that I could achieve alone.

My progress was slow (and very nearly ground to a halt with the early arrival of twins), but determined not to let the athlete's amazing stories remain on my computer for eternity, I continued on, and with the help of many amazing people, completed the book just before the twins' first birthday—three and a half years after the idea for this book (and my daughter) was born.

My stubbornness in seeing this project through aside, this book simply couldn't have been possible without the support of many wonderful people. I have to start by thanking my amazing family. None of this would have been possible without the love and support of my incredible better half, Nick. Thank you. For everything. You are simply the best.

I am eternally grateful to my daughter Maeva, for slowing me down enough to think that writing this book was a good idea in the first place. And to my twins, Leo and Lucas, for sleeping (slightly) better and allowing me to keep pushing away, slowly, at the writing and editing in the tiny windows of availability, night after night. Thank you to my dear mum Sherry, for dutifully and encouragingly reading all of the first, and last, edits. And to my dad Rob, for always believing in me.

To all of my friends, thank you for patiently listening to me talk about this book for what must have seemed like forever during its creation, and for being brave enough to continually ask me how 'the book' was going, especially to those of you with absolutely no interest in knees or sport!

A very special thank you to the ever-patient Geoff Slattery for his wonderful editing skills and publishing experience, and for believing from the start that this book 'had legs'. And to the wise women from the Australian Women Who Write group who answered my many questions in the early stages when I had absolutely no idea what was involved in the process of writing a book: in particular Rachel Oakes-Ash, Claire Halliday, and Sarah Thornton. And to the lovely Michele Smart, for such effervescent enthusiasm and advice in the project's infancy.

I am forever indebted to the keen eyes and vast knowledge base of all of the very clever people who laid eyes on the manuscript—from the early chapter edits through to the final proofs. Thank you to David Joyce, Kay Robinson, Matt Whalan, Kate MacDermid, Lachlan Wilmot, Holly Crawford, Victoria Beattie, Emily Lawrence, Sherry Cunningham, and Andy Bingeman. Shaun Miller, thank you also for your legal expertise, and Alice Beattie for your creative skills in cover design.

To all of the athletes who generously and enthusiastically volunteered their time for an interview, usually conducted at some strange hour around my children's nap schedules, this book wouldn't be possible without your stories. Simply put, your stories ARE the book. Thank you for so openly sharing your lived experiences.

Thank you also to the array of colleagues who helped me to connect with athletes outside my direct working circle—Will Morgan, Alanna Antcliff, Andrew Duff, Sharron Flahive, Sim Freeman, Thihan Chandramohan,

Benny Pagett, Mick Hughes, Dan Mitchell, Randall Cooper.

To the fantastic human who is David Joyce, thank you for being my professional sounding board, and for your ongoing support and encouragement from my first mention of the idea.

To the amazing Ginny Bush, thank you for providing me with a front row seat to so many ACL injuries and their management early in my career. Working with you at Wanaka Physiotherapy, and in particular the on-mountain Snow Park Physio clinic, provided me with the unique experience of seeing ACL injuries happen in real time from the clinic window (often multiple times a day), the opportunity to immediately assess the knees, and then follow up with their rehab and management in the clinic in Wanaka.

Donna White, thank you for your understanding of elite sport's travel requirements, and enabling me to juggle my winter sports work commitments around a busy clinical caseload. Thank you also for your unwavering support during my own physical grievances.

Ashleigh Wolff (née Merkur), thank you for your calm guidance over the years. And to the Olympic Winter Institute of Australia, thank you for all of the incredible opportunities presented to me.

To my phenomenal friend Tori Beattie, thank you for your wonderful friendship, and for the challenges your knee presented me as your therapist. You remain my ongoing inspiration for wanting to ensure the best management and rehab is available to anyone having suffered an ACL injury.

Anna Segal and Russ Henshaw, thank you and your ACL-less knees for inspiring this book (and for the extra grey hairs!)

And finally, to all of the amazing athletes and clients I have had the pleasure of working with over the years; thank you for all that you, your challenges, and your difficult knees, have taught me.

—Jess Cunningham

GLOSSARY

Accessory navicular An extra bone or piece of cartilage located on the inner arch of the foot which is usually asymptomatic, but may become painful if inflamed.

Achilles graft A type of allograft used in ACL reconstruction where an Achilles tendon is obtained from a deceased donor, then sterilised and processed, before being transplanted into the recipient's knee.

ACL—anterior cruciate ligament One of the main stabilising ligaments of the knee that runs diagonally inside the knee joint from the front of the shin bone (tibia) to the back of the thigh bone (femur), forming a cross with the other cruciate ligament - the PCL. It stops the tibia from moving forwards in relation to the femur, as well as providing some rotational control.

Adductor release A surgical procedure that involves cutting/releasing the adductor (groin) muscle tendon where it attaches onto the pubic bone to relieve the tension on the pubic bone and resultant hip/groin/pubic pain and dysfunction.

AFL Auskick An inclusive non-contact junior Australian Rules Football (AFL) development program for ages five to 12.

Allograft—cadaver graft Tissue from a deceased donor that has been sterilised and processed before being transplanted to the recipient. Commonly an Achilles tendon is used for an ACL reconstruction.

Allograft—living donor Tissue from a living donor, such as a hamstring tendon from a parent, that can be used as an ACL graft.

AlterG anti-gravity treadmill A piece of rehabilitation/training equipment that allows the user to walk or run at a lower percentage of their body weight.

Articular cartilage The smooth pearly white tissue that covers the end of bones where they join to form joints. It allows gliding of the surfaces with minimal friction, but can become damaged with injury or overuse.

Atrophy The gradual loss of muscle fibre size and number due to disuse.

Autograft A surgical graft using the person's own tissue. In ACL reconstructions, the graft is commonly taken from the tendon of the hamstring, patella, or quadriceps, and transplanted into the knee.

Avulsion fracture A fracture that occurs when a small chunk or fragment of bone attached to a tendon or ligament gets pulled away from the main part of the bone.

Baker's cyst A fluid-filled sac that causes a bulge and feeling of tightness behind the knee. It occurs when swelling in the knee joint pushes backwards into a bursa (cushioning sac) at the back of the knee.

Bone graft A surgical procedure that uses transplanted bone to repair and rebuild damaged or diseased bone. In recurrent ACL reconstructions, it may be required to plug the bone holes created from the initial surgery, before the subsequent ACL reconstruction can be completed.

Bone spur—osteophyte Bony projections that develop along the edge of bones, commonly in joints, due to degenerative changes.

Cadaver graft—allograft See Allograft

Chondral cartilage See articular cartilage

Closed-chain exercise Any exercise in which the segment furthest from the body is fixed (ie. squat), compared to a closed-chain exercise where the same segment is not fixed (ie. leg extensions).

Cortisone injection An injection of a corticosteroid (a powerful anti-inflammatory medication) used to reduced pain.

CT scan—computerised tomography A medical imaging technology that uses computers and a series of X-ray images from different angles to produce cross sectional images of the body.

Cyst An abnormal fluid filled sac that can develop in tissues in any part in the body.

Dietitian An expert in diet and nutrition. In sport their role is to enhance performance, minimise injury risk, and assist with recovery and healing through advice surrounding nutrition, strategic timing of foods and fluid, and appropriate integration of supplements.

DIN setting The release force setting of a ski binding. It is the value that determines the amount of force needed for a binding to release in order to keep the skier from being injured.

Dislocation An injury where a joint is forced out of its normal position, often due to trauma.

Double-bundled hamstring graft The hamstring graft is folded over to form a two-layered graft, in an effort to make the graft stronger.

Dyno testing A form of muscle testing using specific equipment (isokinetic dynamometer) that measures strength and power of different muscle groups. It can be helpful to highlight differences between the injured and uninjured knee, and muscle imbalances surrounding the injured knee.

Facet joints Pairs of small joints in between the vertebrae at the back of the spine. They allow the spine to bend and twist, and keep the vertebrae from sliding forward, or backwards on one another, or twisting too far. In the lumbar spine they are numbered L1-5, in the thoracic spine T1-12, and the cervical spine C1-7.

Game Ready Performance A medical rehabilitative device that provides hot or cold active compression for injury management and recovery.

Groomers A ski run that has been manicured or 'groomed' by a machine to produce smooth skiing conditions.

Hamstring graft A type of autograft used in ACL reconstruction where the tendon of the semitendinosus hamstring is taken by the surgeon via a small incision over the hamstring attachment to the tibia. The remaining hamstring tissue not taken for the graft is left to heal naturally.

ITB—iliotibial band A long piece of fascia (connective tissue) that runs along the outside of the thigh from the hip to knee and shin bone.

Lachman test A physical examination test used by clinicians to assess the integrity of the ACL ligament.

LARS graft (Ligament Augmentation and Reconstruction System) An artificial ligament used as a synthetic graft for ACL reconstruction.

Lax, laxity Looseness of a tissue that can be genetic in nature or result from over stretching or trauma. Eg. ACL laxity from injury.

LCL—lateral collateral ligament Found on the lateral (outside) side of the knee connecting the tibia to the femur. It stops side to side movement of the knee, particularly varus (bow-legged) forces.

Ligament sprain Grade 1: Ligament has stretched further than normal, but with tearing of fibres and displays minimal laxity; **Grade 2:** Ligament is partially torn, but with some fibres still remaining intact. Displays mild to moderate laxity; **Grade 3:** Ligament is completely torn, with no fibres remaining intact. Displays severe laxity.

MacIntosh loop A surgical procedure that can be used to improve stability in knees with a high degree of rotational instability, or as an addition during ACL revision surgery. It involves using a portion of the iliotibial band to reinforce that lateral aspect of the knee.

MCL—medial collateral ligament Found on the medial (inside) side of the knee connecting the tibia to the femur. It stops side to side movement of the knee, particularly valgus (knock-knee) forces.

Medial meniscectomy A surgical procedure (usually performed arthroscopically) where either the whole, or part of the medial meniscus is removed.

Meningitis Inflammation of the fluid and membranes (meninges) surrounding the brain and spinal cord.

Meniscus A C-shaped pad of cartilage (each knee has two – a medial and lateral meniscus) within the knee that acts as a shock absorber between the femur and tibia, as well as having a roll in knee stability.

Mesh (surgical) A medical device used to provide support to weakened or damaged tissues – commonly used in hernia repairs and other pelvic surgeries.

Microfracture surgery A surgical technique that aims to repair articular cartilage (the cartilage on the end of bones) by creating tiny fractures in the underlying bone (created with a pointed surgical instrument). The subsequent bleeding and clotting from the bone microfractures results in the development of new overlying cartilage.

Mirena IUD (intrauterine device) A hormone (progesterone) releasing intrauterine system that can be used for long-term (up to seven years) birth control and to treat heavy and painful periods.

MRI—magnetic resonance imaging A medical imaging technology that uses a magnetic field and low energy radio waves to produce detailed three-dimensional anatomical images of inside the body.

Navicular A wedge-shaped bone located in the mid foot.

Neuromuscular training program A training program that incorporates general and sport-specific strength and conditioning activities, such as resistance, dynamic stability, balance, core strength, plyometrics and agility exercises to improve performance and prevent injuries. There are many such sport-specific programs available that have been shown to reduce ACL-injury occurrence.

NFL scouting combine A yearly week-long showcase where American college football players undergo physical and mental testing in front of National Football League (NFL) team doctors, coaches, managers, and other performance personnel that allows upcoming draft prospects to be evaluated in a standardised setting.

Nordic hamstring curl A hamstring strengthening exercise that works the hamstrings eccentrically (contracting whilst lengthening). The participant kneels with their feet secured under a stable object and then slowly lowers themselves to the floor keeping their body straight.

Open-chain exercise Any exercise in which the segment furthest from the body is not fixed (ie. leg extensions), compared to a closed-chain exercise where the same segment is fixed (ie. squat).

Osteochondroma A non-cancerous bone growth that develops during childhood or adolescence and forms on the surface of a bone near the growth plate (area of cartilage near the end of bones where new bone growth occurs).

Patella tendon graft A type of autograft used in ACL reconstruction where the middle section of the patella tendon is taken by the surgeon along with small plugs of bone on each end (from where the tendon attaches to the patella and tibia). The remaining patella tendon on either side of the graft site is sutured back together.

Patella tendonitis, patella tendinopathy Inflammation and/or degeneration of the patella tendon (the tendon connecting the kneecap to the shin bone).

Patella tracking The natural movement of the patella on the thighbone as the knee bends and straightens, which can become painful in the presence of muscular imbalances and/or pathology around the knee and hip.

PCL—posterior cruciate ligament The other cruciate ligament that runs diagonally with its counterpart—the ACL—inside the knee joint from the back of the shin bone (tibia) to the front of the thigh bone (femur). It stops the tibia from moving backwards in relation to the femur.

Personal trainer A certified individual with the level of competency for creating and delivering safe and effective exercise programs to healthy or medically cleared individuals.

Physiotherapist, physical therapist An allied health professional who is an expert in the structure of the human body and its movement. They are involved in the assessment, diagnosis, planning, and management of a broad range of health conditions including sports injuries (such as ACL injury) and musculoskeletal conditions, through to chronic health conditions.

PICC line—peripherally inserted central catheter line A long soft catheter (tube) that can be used to deliver medicines for serious infections needing intravenous (IV) antibiotics for a few weeks. It is much longer than a standard IV line, running all the way from the arm, neck, or leg, to the heart.

Pilates reformer A piece of pilates equipment, often used for rehabilitation, that consists of a bed-like frame with a sliding platform attached to springs which provide varied resistance.

Pivot shift test A physical examination test used by clinicians to assess the integrity of the ACL ligament.

Plyometric training A type of exercise that trains muscles to produce power through combining the elements of speed and strength.

Proprioception The sense of self-movement and body position.

PRP—platelet rich plasma therapy A treatment technique that involves injecting a concentrated dose of a patient's own platelets (a type of blood cells involved in clotting and healing) to accelerate the healing of tendons, ligaments, muscles and joints.

Quads, quadriceps Primarily, a group of four muscles that make up the front of the thigh (the 'quads').

Quads tendon graft A type of autograft used in ACL reconstruction where a small partial thickness mid-section of the central quadriceps tendon is taken by the surgeon. Most of the quads tendon is uninvolved.

Scaphoid One of the eight carpal bones located on the thumb side of the wrist.

Scope, arthroscope A minimally invasive surgical procedure used to look inside a joint using a small thin tube with a camera and light attached. The surgeon assesses the joint and guides their surgical instruments by watching the camera's images on a video monitor.

Sports doctor, sports physician A medical practitioner who has gained specialist qualifications in sport and exercise medicine and provides expert diagnosis and management of musculoskeletal injuries.

Sports psychologist A psychologist with specialised training in sports performance who helps teams and athletes to improve their performance, overcome problems, and achieve their goals through use of mental skills and training.

Stem cells Special cells that can develop into different cell types such as muscle, bone, or cartilage cells. Stem cell therapy promotes the repair response of specific cells that have been damaged or lost, such as regenerating damaged cartilage in the knee.

Strength and conditioning coach (S&C) A physical performance professional who uses exercise prescription to improve teams and athletes sporting performance.

Stress fracture Tiny cracks in a bone, most commonly caused by overuse or repetitive activity.

THC and CBD oil Delta-9 Tetrahydrocannabidiol and Cannabidiol Medicinal oil derived from the cannabis plant with reported benefits of reducing pain and inflammation. The CBD compound does not have psychoactive properties, whereas delta-9 tetrahydrocannabinol does.

Tibial osteotomy A surgical procedure that literally means 'cutting of the bone'. A wedge of bone is removed from the tibia (shin bone) to realign the leg and the forces experienced through the knee joint.

Tibial slope The posterior inclination of the tibial plateau. An increased tibial slope is thought to be a contributing factor to ACL injury risk.

VMO – vastus medialis oblique A small component of one of the four quadriceps muscles that sits on the inside of the knee. As well as extending the knee it helps to control and stabilise the patella (knee cap).

Yoyo (beep) test A fitness test that involves running at increasing speeds between markers spaced 20 metres apart until exhaustion.

ENDNOTES

1   Zbrojkiewicz, D, V.C., & Grayson, J.E. (2018). Increasing rates of anterior cruciate ligament reconstruction in young Australians, 2000–2015. *Medical Journal of Australia*, 208(8), 354-358.

2   Hewett, T., Ford, K., Hoogenboom, B., & Myer, G. (2010). Understanding and preventing ACL injuries: Current biomechanical and epidemiologic considerations – Update. *North American Journal of Sports and Physical Therapy*. 5(4), 234-251.

3   Owoeye, O.B.A., VanderWey, M.J. & Pike, I. (2020). Reducing injuries in soccer (football): an umbrella review of best evidence across the epidemiological framework for prevention. *Sports Medicine - Open*, 6(1), 46. doi: 10.1186/s40798-020-00274-7

4   Crossley, K.M., Patterson, B.E., Culvenor, A.G., Bruder, A.M., Mosler, A.B., & Mentiplay, B.F. (2020). Making football safer for women: a systematic review and meta-analysis of injury prevention programmes in 11 773 female football (soccer) players. *British Journal of Sports Medicine*, 54(18),1089-1098. doi: 10.1136/bjsports-2019-101587

5   Webster, K.E., & Hewett, T.E. (2018). Meta-analysis of meta-analyses of anterior cruciate ligament injury reduction training programs. *Journal of Orthopaedic Research*, 36(10), 2696-2708. doi: 10.1002/jor.24043

6   Whalan, M., Lovell, R., Steele, J.R., & Sampson, J.A. (2019). Rescheduling Part 2 of the 11+ reduces injury burden and increases compliance in semi-professional football. *Scandinavian Journal of Medicine and Science in Sports*, 29(12),1941-1951. doi: 10.1111/sms.13532

7   Grindem, H., A.J. Arundale, & C.L. Ardern. (2018). Alarming underutilisation of rehabilitation in athletes with anterior cruciate ligament reconstruction: four ways to change the game. *British Journal of Sports Medicine*, 52(18), 1162-1163. doi: 10.1136/bjsports-2017-098746

8   Ihara, H., & Kawano, T. (2017). Influence of age on healing capacity of acute tears of the anterior cruciate ligament based on magnetic resonance imaging assessment. *Journal of Computer Assisted Tomography*, 41(2), 206-211. doi: 10.1097/RCT.0000000000000515

9   Costa-Paz, M., Ayerza, M. A., Tanoira, I., Astoul, J., & Muscolo, D. L. (2012). Spontaneous healing in complete ACL ruptures: a clinical and MRI study. *Clinical Orthopaedics and Related Research*, 470(4), 979–985. https://doi.org/10.1007/s11999-011-1933-8

10 Fujimoto, E., Sumen, Y., Ochi, M., & Ikuta, Y. (2002). Spontaneous healing of acute anterior cruciate ligament (ACL) injuries - conservative treatment using an extension block soft brace without anterior stabilization. *Archives of Orthopaedic and Trauma Surgery*, 122(4), 212-6. doi: 10.1007/s00402-001-0387-y

11 Filbay, S., Roemer, F., Lohmander, S., Turkiewicz, A., Roos, E.M., Frobell, R., & Englund, M. (2022). Spontaneous healing of the ruptured anterior cruciate ligament: observations from the KANON trial. *BMJ Open Sport & Exercise Medicine*, 8. doi: 10.1136/bmjsem-2022-sportskongres.8

12 Frobell, R.B., Roos, H.P., Roos, E.M., Roemer, F.W., Ranstam, J., & Lohmander, L.S. (2013). Treatment for acute anterior cruciate ligament tear: five year outcome of randomised trial. *BMJ*. 24, 346:f232. doi: 10.1136/bmj.f232

13 Meuffels, D.E., Favejee, M.M., Vissers, M.M., Heijboer, M.P., Reijman, M., & Verhaar, J.A. (2009). Ten year follow-up study comparing conservative versus operative treatment of anterior cruciate ligament ruptures. A matched-pair analysis of high level athletes. *British Journal of Sports Medicine*. 43(5), 347-51. doi: 10.1136/bjsm.2008.049403

14 Grindem, H., Eitzen, I., Moksnes, H., Snyder-Mackler, L., & Risberg, M.A. (2012). A pair-matched comparison of return to pivoting sports at 1 year in anterior cruciate ligament-injured patients after a nonoperative versus an operative treatment course. *American Journal of Sports Medicine*, 40(11), 2509-16. doi: 10.1177/0363546512458424

15 Kovalak, E., Atay, T., Çetin, C., Atay, I.M., & Serbest, M.O. (2018). Is ACL reconstruction a prerequisite for the patients having recreational sporting activities? *Acta Orthopaedia et Traumatologica* Turcica, 52(1), 37-43. doi: 10.1016/j.aott.2017.11.010

16 Weiler, R., Monte-Colombo, M., Mitchell, A. &, Haddad, F. (2015). Non-operative management of a complete anterior cruciate ligament injury in an English Premier League football player with return to play in less than 8 weeks: applying common sense in the absence of evidence. *BMJ Case Reports*, 26, 2015:bcr2014208012. doi: 10.1136/bcr-2014-208012

17 Weiler, R. (2016). Unknown unknowns and lessons from non-operative rehabilitation and return to play of a complete anterior cruciate ligament injury in English Premier League football. *British Journal of Sports Medicine*, 50(5), 261-2. doi: 10.1136/bjsports-2015-095141

18 Keays, S.L., Newcombe, P., & Keays, A.C. (2019). Nearly 90% participation in sports activity 12 years after non-surgical management for anterior cruciate ligament injury relates to physical outcome measures. *Knee Surgery, Sports Traumatology, Arthroscopy*. 27(8), 2511-2519. doi: 10.1007/s00167-018-5258-y

19 Roos, H., Ornell, M., Gärdsell, P., Lohmander, L.S., & Lindstrand, A. (1995). Soccer after anterior cruciate ligament injury--an incompatible combination? A national survey of incidence and risk factors and a 7-year follow-up of 310 players. *Acta Orthopaedica Scandanavica*, 66(2), 107-12. doi: 10.3109/17453679508995501

20 van Yperen, D.T., Reijman, M., van Es, E.M., Bierma-Zeinstra, S.M.A., & Meuffels, D.E. (2018). Twenty-year follow-up study comparing operative versus nonoperative treatment of anterior cruciate ligament ruptures in high-level athletes. *American Journal of Sports Medicine*, 46(5), 1129-1136. doi: 10.1177/0363546517751683

21 Delincé, P., & Ghafil, D. (2012). Anterior cruciate ligament tears: conservative or surgical treatment? A critical review of the literature. *Knee Surgery, Sports Traumatology, Arthroscopy*, 20(1), 48-61. doi: 10.1007/s00167-011-1614-x

22 Smith, T.O., Postle, K., Penny, F., McNamara, I., & Mann, C.J. (2014). Is reconstruction the best management strategy for anterior cruciate ligament rupture? A systematic review and meta-analysis comparing anterior cruciate ligament reconstruction versus non-operative treatment. *Knee*, 21(2), 462-70. doi: 10.1016/j.knee.2013.10.009

23 Monk, A.P., Davies, L.J., Hopewell, S., Harris, K., Beard, D.J., & Price, A.J. (2016). Surgical versus conservative interventions for treating anterior cruciate ligament injuries. *Cochrane Database of Systemic Reviews*, 3;4(4):CD011166. doi: 10.1002/14651858.CD011166.pub2

24 Beischer, S., Gustavsson, L., Senorski, E.H., Karlsson, J., Thomeé, C., Samuelsson, K., & Thomeé, R. (2020). Young athletes who return to sport before 9 months after anterior aruciate ligament reconstruction have a rate of new injury 7 times that of those who delay return. *Journal of Orthopaedics & Sports Physical Therapy*, 50(2), 83-90. doi: 10.2519/jospt.2020.9071

25 Armento, A., Albright, J., Gagliardi, A., Daoud, A.K., Howell, D., & Mayer, S. (2021). Patient expectations and perceived social support related to return to sport after anterior cruciate ligament reconstruction in adolescent athletes. *Physical Therapy in Sport, 47*:72-77. doi: 10.1016/j.ptsp.2020.10.011

26 Toole, A.R., Ithurburn, M.P., Rauh, M.J., Hewett, T.E., Paterno, M.V., & Schmitt, L.C. (2017). Young athletes cleared for sports participation after anterior cruciate ligament reconstruction: How many actually meet recommended return-to-sport criterion cutoffs? *Journal of Orthopaedics & Sports Physical Therapy*, 47(11), 825-833. doi: 10.2519/jospt.2017.7227.

27 Welling, W., Benjaminse, A., Seil, R., Lemmink, K., Zaffagnini, S., & Gokeler, A. (2018). Low rates of patients meeting return to sport criteria 9 months after anterior cruciate ligament reconstruction: a prospective longitudinal study. Knee Surgery, *Sports Traumatology, Arthroscopy*. 26(12), 3636-3644. doi: 10.1007/s00167-018-4916-4